Insomnia and *Stretch to Sleep*™-Program

Insomnia and *Stretch to Sleep*™-Program

Claes Zell

iUniverse, Inc.
Bloomington

INSOMNIA AND *STRETCH TO SLEEP*™-PROGRAM

The information, ideas, and suggestions in this book are not intended as a substitute for professional medical advice. Before following any suggestions contained in this book, you should consult your personal physician. Neither the author nor the publisher shall be liable or responsible for any loss or damage allegedly arising as a consequence of your use or application of any information or suggestions in this book.

iUniverse books may be ordered through booksellers or by contacting:

iUniverse
1663 Liberty Drive
Bloomington, IN 47403
www.iuniverse.com
1-800-Authors (1-800-288-4677)

Because of the dynamic nature of the Internet, any web addresses or links contained in this book may have changed since publication and may no longer be valid. The views expressed in this work are solely those of the author and do not necessarily reflect the views of the publisher, and the publisher hereby disclaims any responsibility for them.

Any people depicted in stock imagery provided by Thinkstock are models, and such images are being used for illustrative purposes only.

Certain stock imagery © Thinkstock.

ISBN: 978-1-4759-7997-8 (sc)
ISBN: 978-1-4759-7998-5 (hc)
ISBN: 978-1-4759-7999-2 (e)

Library of Congress Control Number: 2013905097

Printed in the United States of America

iUniverse rev. date: 3/18/2013

Contents

Preface

I had sleeping problems most of my early life. When I moved from home as a young man, it got worse, which had a very negative impact on my daily life, both at work as a postman and later when I studied at the Royal Institute of Technology. When needed a healthy sleep, I mostly had to cope with sleeping less than half the time. In the beginning of the 1990s, I started to use stretching techniques, mainly to release leg stiffness. Immediately, I felt their benefits for the quality of my sleep as well.

Sports and physical activities have always been on the agenda for me, and therefore, the step to study massage techniques was not a big one. My interests for human body took me to a journey in alternative medicine for many years. Later on, to broaden my education and to fit to KAM, committee for alternative medicine, roles I study traditional medicine. This was a special course for alternative therapist and I received an education degree in medicine at Uppsala University Biomedical Center. After a quarter of a century of experience with my self-devised stretching techniques, I thought it would be great to share them with other sufferers, because sleep is so important in every aspect of human life. I started to investigate why I had been helped so much by my stretching techniques. Many years of interest in medicine gave me the opportunity to research from vast sources of information. I assemble my thoughts and ideas from many years of experiences and self-made techniques, all of which have helped to improve my sleep.

There are many reasons for bad sleep, but with this book, I want to help improve your sleep—without medicine, using easy-to-learn techniques that require only the effort of your own time.

Acknowledgments

Personal thanks to friends and associates

To talk to a friend when you feel for it, or need it, it is always precious. To write a book it is quite a task and to receive support now and then lifts you up. -If you can't take a risk in life you don't achieve or win anything; many successful risks taker claim. Never theless, I have a bunch of friends to thank.

First of all, I want to thank Pauline. You always believed in me and from the start had confidence in my book project. -Meeting you gave me strength to write directly into English, instead of using my native language Swedish. Thanks for your love and support.

Peter, my brother and his wife, Gull, have been bombarded with thoughts and theories many years in the past. Sometimes, having the nearest family as an objective advice panel is not always the right medium, never the less, thanks for all your help and patience.

Ingrid, you gave me strength in the second half of this book. You said on one occasion, gathered together with a bunch of friends, that you admired my courage and goal-oriented mind and that I still stick to my plan despite delays. Even a little chat at a party gives positive vibrations for quite some time. Thanks for your nice words.

Jon, you have shown great interest in my book and kept asking me how the project was coming along. Thanks for your concern.

Alex and Pia, we had a couple of hours together in yours summer house. We discussed my project very late in the process and you two gave me full support and hoped for the best. Thanks, that was a nice gesture.

Douglas A., you gave me the opportunity to start my book project at the very beginning. You said that you believed in my idée and plans, and you gave me the important starting energy.

Insomnia and *Stretch to Sleep*™-Program

Fredrik S., we have had good talks several times throughout the process, about writing a book and the key issues. Since you already wrote your first one, you have quite some experience in the field. Thanks for your support.

Lasse B., you read my manuscript just in the end of the final results, with great interest and gave me valuable comments and improved the manuscript.

Mats S., we have had continued communications throughout my whole project, which gave me a robust platform to hold on to. Thanks for your support.

Maria O., Thanks for all your help and patience regarded new illustrations for my book.

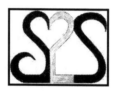

Introduction

In the process of writing this book, I talked to a friend and said, "I am working on a book about sleep and sleep problems." There was a moment of silence, and then he asked, "Why?" He sincerely didn't have a clue why a book needed to be written. "Take a deep breath, put your head on a pillow, relax, and sleep," he said in a very confident voice.

How do you reply to that? And where do you start? Unfortunately, the consensus among the public and my own experience tell me it's not that easy. If you don't have any opinion or interest about your own sleep, then surely you must gain a sufficient number of sleeping hours. You don't think about it. You don't need to. Nevertheless, for all the sufferers out there, almost 30 percent (enough for me), I wrote this book.

Over the last couple of decades we seem to have gained a lesser quality of sleep, and we generally don't get enough sleeping hours. The main problem seems to be our lack of ability to calm down at the end of the day. Our top priority is to find something quick and easy to use whenever we can't fall asleep. If we look at our society and the progress in the last couple hundred years, is it strange that we can't relax on demand? No, I don't think so! Modern man has experienced and achieved a lot, but who has paid? Technical success and the development of science have taken their toll. We have lost our ability to relax, and without the gift of cooling down, you can't sleep. For some, these skills are natural, but unfortunately, not for all of us.

Is there a method for those people struggling for better sleep? Yes, I think there is. Is there a method simple enough for everybody use? Yes, I think so. But, it's a time and labor issue. You have to make some effort, reasonable short time, to make this to happen. As I explain further on some people are prone to store stress in their bodies and that is my key task to dissolve that stress. People with poor sleep can't have any form of out coming disruption and weak sleep abilities craving all forms of solutions. My S2S-program can be yours main sleep solution to better sleep.

Increased Stress Level

It has been a spectacular journey for the human race, with 250 years of rapid improvement of almost everything you can imagine. Fast-paced technological innovations and population growth have occurred in a very short period of time. However, do we understand how much everything has increased during the last century and how big its impact is in our lives according to our stress levels? You can look at the numbers below. Regardless of your opinion of some of these points, they're still interesting to look at and can make you think ahead about where we are going in the future.

The Industrial Revolution

In the Second Industrial Revolution, beginning around 1850, technological and economic progress took a massive leap with the development of steam-powered ships and railways. Historians agree that this period was one of the most important events in history. From the end of the nineteenth century, we have had tremendous development for almost everything we can measure. This Second Industrial Revolution, known also as the Technological Revolution, has had a major impact on mankind, and also people's stress levels. In the long run, this Technological Revolution has brought economic improvement for mankind in industrialized societies.

One of the major technological impacts in the last century was the revolutionary invention of computers and mobile phones. Nowadays, telephones are essential, and everybody (even small children) has mobile phones. But in the time of Alexander Graham Bell, communication among people must have been very different. Alexander Graham Bell (1847–1922) was an eminent scientist, engineer, and innovator; he got a US patent for the first practical telephone in 1876. The fact that his mother and wife were deaf profoundly influenced Bell's lifework of understanding the exchange of information and also he had a father and grandfather who were dedicated to speech-related issues, as well. Bell's telephone must have been one of the most important innovations for speeding up the Industrial Revolution in the end of the 1900s, but despite these genius applications, Bell wasn't keen to use the

14

telephone himself, due to interruption issues. He simply thought he didn't have time to answer the phone during the daytime. What on earth would he have felt about our modern days of hectic life? We will never know, but he must have suspected the revolutionary influences that would result from his own genius invention of the telephone.

Environmental changes

Environmental changes, which are not scientific proven, in the last century include:

Increased:

- Sound levels 200 times
- Information flood 10,000 times
- Electric radiation 1 million times

Decreased:

- Body movement 20 times
- Nourishment 15 times

I picked those figures up years ago but I still think they are interesting to look at, although knowing that some might be incorrect. Everybody knows all these environmental parameters have been changing, tremendously, the last 250 years. The two world wars have had a big impact on the industrial war trade and business. The computer and the TV age have been boosted with never-ending electricity and resulted in information floods. Our bodies seem to be trapped within more and more external input, and external intruders of all kinds are what insomnia sufferers cannot handle.

The Industrial Revolution has continued over several generations, but it has been clearly shown that something is happening or changing lately. It can't be coincidence! The statistics, for instance Swedish Statistics (SCB/ULF), of insomnia outbreak are very clear, and they are now at a peak, growing continuously since the period of

1991-1992. Look for yourself. The five environmental changes noted above, you must agree, have had major impact on our sleep. Just consider the electrification of our society since 150 years ago and the starting of computerization in the last quarter of the previous century. '

Twenty-first-century syndrome

Twenty-first-century syndrome, or the adrenal fatigue syndrome, is a term first coined in 1998 by Dr. James Wilson (2002), a Canadian alternative medicine specialist. The syndrome is quite a new name and did not get accepted everywhere in the medical establishment. Twenty-first-century syndrome involves the following:

- Little exercise
- Unhealthy foods
- Complex metabolic disorders

William Dement, a professor of psychiatry at Stanford University, found that there is a correlation between sleep and health. He said: "In maintaining good health, sleep may be more critical than diet, exercise, and even heredity." He and his associates measured cognitive abilities, memory, and motor skills after sleep deprivation and found that those who regularly missed sleep became more or less intoxicated. This has also been shown through experiments on animals: mice that have slept enough but ate poorly, lived longer, in comparison to overeating mice with minimum sleeping hours—a classic scenario of obesity! After only four hours of sleep, the body has difficulty regulating blood sugar. Therefore, the body compensates the energy loss by releasing hormones to make up for the lack of energy—reducing leptin in blood plasma and increasing the amount of ghrelin. This compensation creates a strong craving for heavier carbohydrates. To sleep less makes you eat more and gain more weight; in some people, it causes obesity.

If you eat over your limit of carbohydrates, you're risking stabilizing a high level of insulin, and this might end up in a fatal future scenario of a bunch of life-threatening conditions. Ghrelin has an important influence on nerves, particularly in the hippocampus, and is essential for cognitive adaptation and the process of learning, among other processes.

Plamen Penev, MD, PhD, University of Chicago, stated from a small study: "Among other hormonal effects, we found that sleep restriction caused an increase in ghrelin levels in the blood. Ghrelin is a hormone that has been shown to reduce energy, stimulate hunger and food intake, promote retention of fat, and increase glucose production in the body. This could explain why sleep-deprived participants also reported feeling hungrier during the study."

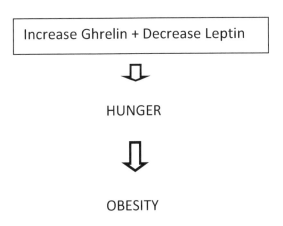

Figure 1. Sleep-deprivation effects

Glucose-PET studies have shown that after twenty-four hours of sustained wakefulness, sleep deprivation results mainly in the decrease of immune system function and growth hormones.

The functions of many organ systems are also linked to the sleep cycle, for instance, the endocrine system. Sleep is one of the events that modify the timing of secretion for certain hormones. Many hormones are secreted into the blood during sleep. Scientists believe that the release of growth hormone is related to repair processes that occur during sleep. Other hormones released during sleep are follicle hormone (maturational process) and luteinizing hormone (reproductive process).

Stressful future

Results from an animal study (C. Westenbroeka et al.) show that exposure to chronic stress prevented normal weight gain in both male and female rats. The rats were under intense stress twice daily for fifteen days. Researchers also found that the levels of the stress hormone corticosterone were much higher in female rats exposed to chronic stress than in male rats. Corticosterone is released by the adrenal glands in response to stress in the same pattern that the stress hormone cortisol is released in humans.

Constant stress at work or at home may be more dangerous for women than men, as the rats' study suggested and the opposite according to modern myths about women's abilities to cope with stress; there is a myth that the modern woman can work double-time to achieve the perfect home and raise children without being harmed by stress. Fortunately, this situation is changing to better equalization of the parenting load in many countries. Still, it's important to think about your stress level on a regular basis. Exercise could be one solution, and focusing on your mental and physical health can put you at an advantage later in life. Exposure to high levels of these stress hormones can lead to a bigger waistline, which is a major risk factor of heart disease, and a decreased immune system.

There are different ways to look at stress. Minor stress can be defined as acute stress over only a few hours. Major stress can last over days or weeks. Doctors use the medical term *cumulative stress* to describe daily stress over time. That means the increasing effects of daily doses of what we eat and drink, smoking habits, quality of sleep, and so on. Despite the bad connotations of stress, acute stress (short term stress) seems to boost immune function and improve memory. Chronic stress, on the other hand, has the opposite effect and can make your body more open for diseases that are frequent with aging, such as depression, diabetes, and cognitive impairment.

Underlying defects in stress responses and reactions to stress affect patients' brain aging via hormonal effects. According to doctors, depressive illness over a long period of time leads to shrinkage of the hippocampus. The hippocampus belongs to the limbic system for long-term memory and cognitive navigation. In some results, mental stress showed a nearly 30 percent decline of blood flow to the brain. Also, doctors talk more and more about the severity of stress and its influence on heart disease. According to researcher David S. Sheps, MD, MSPH, stress-induced reduction in blood flow to the heart is more common than previously believed. Several studies by the University of Florida research team indicated mental stresses were among the most important risk factors for death in heart patients. One study showed that for some patients, mental stress is as dangerous as smoking cigarettes or having high cholesterol. Scientists are not sure if chronically stressed peoples are less likely to have healthy lifestyles, or if people with unhealthy habits tend to feel more stressed at work. To be aware of your own stress, you should consider your lifestyle every day.

Everybody knows that stress normally has a negative effect on sleep. I wrote "normally" due to the fact that there is such a thing as "positive stress." Positive stress means a state of mind when you act according to your purpose and goal both physically and mentally; you are doing something you can handle and that you like. With positive stress, time flies. You don't have control over the time scale. The time dimension seems to vanish. You work in a hole or a vacuum. All your senses focus only on one specific thing. You work in a flow state, over which you have control. Those times are something positive and will act according to your body and mind. This period of positive stress doesn't have any negative effect; you normally sleep with a smile on your face, thinking or dreaming of the next day's escapades, even if you worked more than the normal number of working hours.

I met an artist, an oil painter, in a gallery in Stockholm on the first day of his exhibition week. After we spent awhile talking about his work, he asked me if I painted as well. I explained that I used to paint—although I was an amateur—but at that moment I was finishing a book.

"What about?" he replied.

"It's about sleeping issues," I told him.

"I have no problem at all," he continued.

Just before going to sleep each night, he would think a moment about what he been doing during the day and whether he needed to change anything the next day. Then he would sleep peacefully, with no concerns about his work. He lived a typically good life. He had total control over his work. He was his own boss. He made the decisions.

But in his early life, though, when he started painting, it was different. He had to struggle to make everything come together, mainly his financial situation and taking care of his children.

Individuals in stressful situations commonly experience difficulty in sleeping, and this can occur in almost anyone in response to acute stressors, such as illness, personal conflict, work-related stress, environmental factors, and sudden schedule changes. Is there any association between stress and insomnia? In a prospective study of young adults assessed over a seven-year period, those who experienced more frequent negative life events and interpersonal conflicts were more likely to have occasional insomnia or repeated periods of brief insomnia.

A Finnish study by Martikainen and associates found that psychosocial stressors were more likely to be associated with insomnia than health problems were, indicating the strong link between stressors and sleep problems. A Japanese study by Utsugi and associates reported that high job stress was associated with a higher risk for insomnia, suggesting that work-related stress may contribute to a combination of both insomnia and sleep deprivation. In a study by Vignau and associates of French adolescents, those who had insomnia symptoms came from families with higher divorce rates, had poorer relationships with their families, and reported higher rates of medical and psychological illness or death in their parents.

Two friends of mine, a young couple who were parents of a beautiful daughter, struggled with a stressful life. One could write a book on this subject of being a parent. Your schedule during this time of life is upside down. Nothing is what it used to be. Taking care of a baby is like going from driving an old rusty car to driving an F1 racer. The collaboration between the young couple needed to be trimmed together tightly. And if you added even more struggle and stressors, they could find things going out of hand. For a young mother with all new hormones pumping in her body, good sleep is like a healing session. This situation is hard to crack almost every time. There is no time for contemplation, no time of the parents' own. A screaming baby and a constant lack of sleep is what many parents have to cope with. Luckily for most parents, this situation gets better in time.

A Swedish study by Linton found that a poor psychosocial work environment led to a more than twofold increased risk for the development of a new episode of insomnia, compared with normal sleepers. Insomnia shows increases in metabolic rate, body temperature, and heart rate. Insomniacs also exhibit higher levels of cortisol, suggesting increased activity of the stress-response system. Poor sleepers also have a significantly higher heart rate. These data suggest that individuals show consistent sleep responses to stressors, and that those with greater sympathetic nervous system activation may be more susceptible to developing insomnia. The results demonstrated that it may be possible to detect vulnerability to insomnia and that such vulnerability is associated with hyperarousal. Arousal levels at bedtime mediated the relationship between stress during the day and sleep disturbance the following night. These findings are not only consistent with physiologic studies of insomnia, but they also suggest that treatment for insomnia should include training in stress management and better coping strategies because an individual's response to stress, doctor's propos. Fortunately, that is what this book is all about: to make a strategic plan for better control of the arousal level and to find the switch to close down hyperactivity in your body, in other words, to change the nervous system activity.

People respond to stress in different ways. Some researchers believe that you should take the internal environment into more consideration than the external. The same stress can affect different humans in different ways; for some, it can produce stress, while it produces happiness for others. The solution to stress lies not in management of external events and situations, but in self-management. "It is difficult to find happiness in oneself, but it is impossible to find it anywhere else," said Arthur Schopenhauer, a German philosopher.

When mental stress raises the blood pressure, it may be a risk factor for hypertension. Blood pressure rises during times of mental stress, but the change varies in level from patient to patient. "If a patient experiences more than a 20 percent increase in blood pressure due to mental stress, there is an abnormal activation of the sympathetic nervous system that could be damaging to blood vessels and vital organs," said Dr. Ingaramo, MD, at the American Society of Hypertension's Twentieth Annual Scientific Meeting. Mental stress could thus be associated with organ damage.

Periods of stressful times can influence the wrong nervous system, and for people with poor sleep, they can be devastating. To better control the nervous system is crucial, and to have the key to do that is a number one priority. But often it is very hard to change the nervous system when you really need to do it. To understand the necessity of switching between the two nervous systems, we have to understand their differences. The golden rule is to close down the sympathetic nervous system and to boost, for the poor sleeper, the parasympathetic system, the "night" system. In the next chapter, I will give you a summary of the most important information to know about your body's nervous system

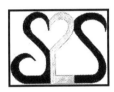

Part 1

Sleep

Sleep is important for all people. Without sleep, we can't function properly. All people have various sleeping needs. Some prefer mornings; others prefer late evenings or nights. We all need a number of sleeping hours each night, and without doubt, sleep quality also has a major importance. The needs of sleep apply in many theories, one of which is the possible connection between sleep and learning in humans. A 2009 study by Peyrache and associates suggests that sleep quality (in terms of deep-sleep hours) has a large impact on learning abilities, based on the electrophysiological recordings of a large number of isolated cells in the prefrontal cortex of rats. The study revealed that the cells that formed upon learning were more active during subsequent sleep episodes. This means that those replay events were more prominent during slow-wave sleep and were coacting with the hippocampus events.

Is sex more important than sleep? I read about a survey not long ago. Sleep is important, we know that. But is it more important than sex? Some of you may say, "Absolutely not!" But what do men think about this issue? Well, a survey clearly showed that 80 percent of British men preferred a good night's sleep, than to be interrupted with a close encounter with their mates. This is surely not due to lack of lust, which is the problem. Sex is just not at the top of the list; many other things have to be taken care of during the day, researchers say.

A major contribution to improving your sleep is how you prepare yourself. Are you still tense and stressed despite several hours having passed since you stopped working for the day? Of course, late evenings for morning people are a bad habit. But those people who like to wake up early in the morning used to go to bed in time in the evening. It is more likely that if you stay up late in the evening, you're doing it because you can't sleep at the right time. This can have a lot of different causes. However, scientists agree that sleep quality is more important than the total number of sleeping hours and that sleep requirements fluctuate from person to person.

Sleep Positions

There are some issues based on sleeping in different positions. Through the years, you have obviously determined your favorite sleep position and you will not sleep in a position that feels unpleasant. My experience, though, is that your favorite sleeping positions may change through the years. I always slept, in my younger years, on my belly, with my left leg drawn up. This used to be called the recovery position. Nowadays, I lie flat on my back, without snoring hopefully. And snoring, unfortunately, is not dealt with in this book. Snoring is normally about a physical throat problem, which needs a lot of medical attention. But what you do in the different sleep stages is harder to do something about. Science states that sleep postures have both negative and positive factors.

You must have heard many times that someone woke up with pain somewhere, mostly in the neck, and said, "I've been sleeping in the wrong position," or something similar.

Belly Position

The belly position, or front position, is sleeping with the legs mostly straight and flat against the bed. This position will help for breathing problems, but you can find comments against this position due to head issues. The head-body junction can be in a strained momentum; that front position can lead to nerve problems in the upper body. Make sure that your cervical vertebrae are not put out of alignment with the spine. This is even more important for older people and for those with increased risk for arthritis conditions.

Half-Side Position

Sleeping in the half-side position used to be described as the "recovery position," because it's similar to the posture used in emergency situations. The main factor is to recover or restore the breathing option. Also, if you have trouble with a medical condition known as gastroesophageal reflux disease, you should sleep on your left side. Sleeping on the right side gave longer recovery from draining out of the esophagus, as compared to sleeping on the left side. Patients felt more discomfort sleeping on that side. It has also been suggested that the sleep-side posture can cause more wrinkles on that side of the face.

Side Position

This is one of the popular position, seven of ten sleepers use this position, and is also called the fetal position. You lie on one side, on your shoulder, with legs more or less drawn up toward your belly. There are some key areas, checkpoints, to consider. What is important in the side position is to have your spine in a straight position; this is often what bed fabricants mention to sell their products. The neck is the other area to look at in this position. The neck and the spine should be in the same horizontal line to be optimal and not give any pain or complaint when waking up. Even so, to have the legs toward the belly gives a release, by curling the body inward, opening up the back, and reducing pressure on the discs. A too-soft bed makes the spine curve down, according to gravitational pull.

Back Position

Sleeping on your back is often used at some time during the night. A well-known factor is that these positions aggravate snoring and sleep apnea. The muscles in the jaw and tongue are relaxed and are pulled down by gravity. Nevertheless, the back position has good influences for distributing weight throughout the body. Research has shown that those who sleep on their backs are more likely to have decreased oxygen levels in their bloodstream, which is a particular concern in patients with heart and circulatory problems. On the other hand, the back position can help give you relief for your tired legs after standing or running about at work. To put a pillow under your legs can switch the nervous system. There is, however, something to bear in mind

Sleep Architecture

You might think that an active life should balance a calm and inactive brain during sleep. In fact, the first third of sleep is a deep state of sleep and there is not much going on; the brain waves are not very active. But after the first part of the sleep cycle, it's the opposite. A Harvard Medical School professor and researcher, J. Allan Hobson, stated that this nightly process accounts for the varied shifts in brain activity throughout the night, resulting in changes in body temperature, chemistry, and sensory activities. The whole function of sleep has not been completely understood, and the absolute hours of necessary sleep are still unknown. The fact is that the human species have a lot in common, but each is still very unique. So when some individuals show full effectiveness with only four to five hours of sleep, others need eight hours of sleep (or even more) to perform at their best.

To measure the animal kingdom sleep habits, you will find that pigs have exactly the same sleeping hours in general as humans, eight hours. But what can we learn from that information, probably nothing. Except that pigs eat in general the same food, a variety of everything, as humans. As more meat you eat more rest/sleep you seems to need, according to animals. And the opposite is; no meat, eat around the clock.

What is probably accurate is that the more quality sleeping hours you get, the more refreshed you feel. Sometimes I think, "How can I feel refreshed when I slept fewer hours than usual?" I have also noticed that if you can't remember waking up in the night, you probably had a good night's sleep without any major breaks. Quality sleep before length of sleep! But there are obviously a lot of parameters to take under consideration.

The knowledge of sleep was described for the first time in the previous century. Lee Loomis provided the earliest detailed description of various stages of sleep in the mid-1930s. With the technique of electroencephalography (EEG), he discovered in 1937 "the sleep K-complex," a typical waveform that occurs in stage 2 sleep. Aserinsky and Kleitman (1955) identified rapid eye movement (REM) sleep. There can be a misconception about sleep, due to its calm and relaxing appearance, but during EEGs you find that sleep isn't a passive and constant state; in fact, it's quite the contrary. Sleep consists of different phases, which are revealed in EEG monitoring, although EEG monitoring has other purposes than to explore sleep, for instance, when it is to discover Alzheimer's plaque in the brain. Both the brain and the body are active during sleep, and the brain is (in some sense) even more active during sleep. The more common (these figures have some variations through medical establishment) brain waves revealed in an EEG are the following:

~ Beta waves, normal awake state: 12–30 Hz
~ Alpha waves, relaxed with closed eyes: 8–12 Hz
~ Theta waves, REM sleep: 6–10 Hz
~ Slow-wave, Delta Sleep: 0.1–4 Hz

Hypnogram

Hypnogram show simplified sleep depths and sleep stages. Every stage represents brain waves (Hz) of a specific category, and a hypnogram is easily describes as a step-by-step diagram. Originally it was based on a set of visual sleep stage scoring rules, which classified the sleep as wakefulness, rapid eye movement (REM) sleep, non-REM sleep stages S1 (lightest sleep) to S4 (deepest sleep), and movement time (MT). Normally a sleep session has six periods, and the first two periods of three hours each contain deep sleep, which you do not often wake up from. If you wake up, it's often after the deep sleep state, and then you can experience or feel overheated. Then REM sleep takes over. At first it may not feel so prominent, but as the night goes by, the sleep gets lighter and REM sleep more characteristic. Hypnogram also reveal specific steps between every stage.

The two major sleep patterns

There are clearly physiological differences between the two major sleep patterns, NREM and REM. NREM sleep represents the calming and rebuilding phase, and REM sleep is the total opposite, which can be seen belove It has been shown (Van Cauter,

28

Leproult) that sleep—more specifically, slow-wave sleep (SWS)—does affect growth hormone levels in adult men. During eight hours' sleep, studies show that the men with a high percentage of SWS (average 24 percent) also had high growth hormone secretion, while subjects with a low percentage of SWS (average 9 percent) had low growth hormone secretion. And we know that growth hormone is extremely important for many processes in your body, for instance, stimulate growth, cell production and regeneration.

The two major sleep patterns:

Physiological Process	During NREM	During REM
Brain Activity	Decrease	Increase
Heart Rate	Decrease	Increase
Blood Pressure	Decrease	Increase

Table 1. Physiological process

Through EEG findings, it's possible to divide sleep into different parts or stages. Doctors normally divide sleep into two main rubrics, which have totally opposite effects toward the human body:

1. Non-rapid eye movement (NREM) sleep

2. Rapid eye movement (REM) sleep

Non-Rapid Eye Movement (NREM) Sleep

What can you find from the name? Non-rapid eye movement sleep is about sleep without rapid eye movement. NREM sleep represents the main part of the sleep

29

cycle, normally 70 to 80 percent of the total sleep time. In the beginning of the period, you'll find the deepest sleep; this is probably the most important period in terms of the renewal processes of the body system. REM sleep represents a very light sleep, with paralytic muscles due to a very hectic dream phase. Without the paralysis state, you would "live out" the dream. In some cases, people do live out the dream, and unfortunately that is not the purpose.

The basal forebrain, including the hypothalamus, is an important region for controlling NREM sleep and may be the region keeping track of how long we have been awake and how large our sleep debt is. The brainstem region known as the pons is important for induced REM sleep. During REM sleep, the pons sends signals to the visual nuclei of the thalamus and to the cerebral cortex, which is responsible for most of our thought processes. The pons also sends signals to the spinal cord, causing the temporary paralysis that is characteristic of REM sleep. Other brain sites are also important in the sleep process. For example, the thalamus generates many of the brain rhythms in NREM sleep that we see as EEG patterns.

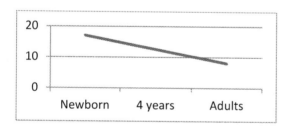

Figure 2. Sleep hours in humans

Newborns sleep an average of seventeen hours per day. By the time a child is three to five years old, total sleep time averages twelve hours a day, and then it further decreases to eight hours per night by adulthood. One of the most prominent age-related changes in sleep is a reduction in the time spent in the deepest stages of NREM (stages 3 and 4) from childhood through adulthood.

The real functions of NREM sleep remain unknown, but one (Benington and Heller) theory proposes a decreased metabolic demand of glycogen stores. This state is shown by PET (positron emission tomography) camera studies, which show that the blood flow decreases throughout the entire brain. As NREM stages progress, stronger stimuli are required to result in an awakening.

NREM sleep stages

During more than half a century, ever since Loomis in 1937, there has been research done on the character of brain waves, according to different sleep stages. There is clearly an oscillation of brain waves through the entire life span, like the heart is beating to supply blood through all the areas of our body. In an awake state, the brain shows alpha waves with electromagnetic oscillations in the frequency range of 8 to 12 Hz.

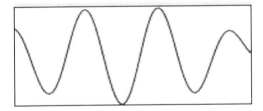

Figure 3. 0.2-second alpha wave

Alpha waves are reduced with closed eyes, drowsiness, and sleep. The most widely researched stage is during the relaxed mental state, where the person is at rest with eyes closed, but is not tired or asleep. The mature alpha wave, at ten waves per second, is firmly established by age.

Alpha waves are common during meditation. You sit with your eyes closed and usually with your legs crossed. The major difference between alpha waves and meditation is that you maintain clearness. You don't want to sleep. Almost twenty years ago, I had a period of half a year where I was very dedicated to meditation. I woke up at four o'clock in the morning and sat for one and a half hours.

Stage **1**

In this stage, sleep is at a state of unconsciousness, in which the brain is relatively more responsive to internal than external stimuli. The brain gradually becomes less responsive to visual, auditory, and other environmental stimuli during the transition from wakefulness to sleep, which is mostly considered as stage 1 of sleep. Slow rolling eye movements (SREM) are usually the first evidence of drowsiness seen on an EEG. This movement is most often horizontal but can also be vertical or oblique. This stage is referred to drowsiness or presleep and is the first or earliest stage of sleep. It is considered to be a transition between wakefulness and sleep. It usually accounts for 2 to 5 percent of total sleep time. If you can't sleep for some reason, this stage increases in duration. And it will also do so as you get older, unfortunately.

Stage 2

This stage is the predominant sleep stage during a normal night's sleep and occurs throughout the sleep period; it represents 45 to 55 percent of total sleep time. The dominant feature in an EEG that establishes stage 2 sleep is the appearance of "sleep spindles" and the K complex.

Both the K-complex and delta wave activity in stage 2 sleep create slow-wave (0.8 Hz) oscillation and delta (1.6–4.0 Hz).

During sleep, these spindles are seen in the brain as bursts of activity immediately following muscle twitching. Researchers think the brain, particularly in the young, is learning about what nerves control what specific muscles when asleep. Also, spindles generated in the region of the thalamus have been shown to aid sleeping in the presence of disruptive external sounds (Dang Vu et. al). Sleep spindle activity has furthermore been found to be associated with the integration of new information into existing knowledge (Tamminen et. al).

Stages 3 and 4

Stage 3 and stage 4 are usually grouped together as slow-wave sleep, SWS, and "delta" sleep. SWS is present more in the first third of the night, and is present when delta waves account for more than 20 percent of the sleep EEG. The difference between stage 3 and stage 4 is only a quantitative matter of the amount of delta activity. When delta activity represents more than 20 to 50 percent of the time you sleep, you are considered to be in stage 3; delta activity is greater than 50 percent of the time when you are in deep 4 stage.

Females in their thirties and forties have been shown to have more delta wave activity than normally, with men showing greater age-related reductions in delta wave activity than females. Delta waves have been shown to decrease across the lifespan, with most of the decline seen in the mid-forties. By the age of about 75, stage four sleep and delta waves may be entirely absent (Colrain et. al).

Delta activity stimulates the release of several hormones including growth hormone releasing hormone GHRH and prolactin (PRL).

Rapid Eye Movement (REM) Sleep

Can you imagine? Around 1.5 kg brain tissues need almost double the blood flow during REM sleep, and we really don't know for sure why we dream. Isn't that strange? We dream very complex scenarios and do things "we just can dream about," so to speak. We do a vast amount of astonishing performances every day on our planet, but we don't need double blood flow for it! The whole Industrial Revolution didn't need double blood flow during the daytime. There must be more to come from scientists in the future on this subject, don't you think? And it has been said for a long time by alternative scientists and spiritual teachers that we use just 10 percent of our brain capacity in general. I know that my teacher in medicine twenty years ago commented on that issue. He said, "If we don't use all our brain tissues, it will be hard to know what we don't use." The main areas of our brain have been identified, and it would therefore be difficult to add nine tenths more. I can agree on that statement. But bear in mind that our universe primarily consists of so-called "black matter," which scientists didn't have a clue about not so long ago (1932).

REM sleep represents 20 to 25 percent of total sleep, and occurs four to five times during a normal eight-hour sleep period. The first REM periods are shorter and will be extended during the rest of the night. To define sleeping stages in a strict way, you have to use polysomnography. Compared to adults, newborns spend far more time in the REM stage; about 50 percent of their total sleep time is REM sleep. In fact, infants fall asleep directly into REM sleep. By two years of age, REM sleep accounts for 20 to 25 percent of total sleep time, which remains relatively constant throughout the remainder of life.

REM sleep is defined by the following:

- Rapid eye movements

- Muscle atonia

Insomnia and *Stretch to Sleep*™-Program

Rapid Eye Movement

If you not have seen it, this state of sleep is quite a play. To truly experience this state, you have to stay awake and look at a sleeping person. The person in REM sleep can give a really active and awake appearance. The body, or rather the major muscles, is in an atonic state, but a person's speech can be very real (if not atonic). If the person suddenly woke up, it would be easy to start talking to him or her, because the speech can be so real, you might think that the person is awake. But after a while, when you haven't received any answer back, you realize that the person is dreaming. And when you look at the person's eyes, you know why the state is named rapid eye movement. I can assure you that these moves are really fast and that the brain is very active; you can clearly see that the person is not in a relaxed state.

The duration of REM sleep increases with each cycle; it tends to dominate late in the sleep period into early morning. Surely you have experienced that at some time; you wake up occasionally (especially during a weekend) with a dream experience, and you can fall into that dream stage again. Researchers believe that REM sleep is involved in brain development, in humans and in most other species.

Muscle Atonia

Rapid eye movement (REM) sleep is the sleep stage during which dreaming occurs. REM sleep also involves paralysis of major muscles; this atonia of muscles results from the active inhibition of motor activity. Therefore, during REM sleep, the release of the neurotransmitters norepinephrine, serotonin, and histamine is completely suppressed. As a result, motor neurons are not stimulated, a condition known as REM atonia. This prevents dreams from resulting in dangerous movements of the body. Sometimes you find, in general, an accelerated respiration. Common REM characteristics include a sense of temporary paralysis upon awakening and hallucinations, visual or auditory, during the transition from sleep to being awake or the opposite.

Surely, you must have been experienced that yourself. Anyway, I have found myself trapped in a dream state more times than I found comfortable. I mean, knowing that you are in a dream state, in an unpleasant one, and can't call for help. But even in that, you do know it is only a dream.

PET studies also show that during REM sleep, blood flow increases in the thalamus. The thalamus plays an important role in regulating states of sleep and wakefulness, and also has a major role in regulating arousal, the level of awareness, and activity. The increase in blood flow to the primary visual regions of the cortex may explain the vivid nature of REM dreaming, while the continued decrease in blood flow to the prefrontal cortex may explain the unquestioning acceptance of even the most bizarre dream content. REM sleep predominates in the last third of the night. A regular night's sleep consists of six periods, and the last two have more REM than the others. REM sleep in infants represents a larger percentage of the total sleep at the expense of stage 3. Until age three to four months, newborns transition from waking directly into REM sleep. In newborns, sleep cycles are very different and last approximately sixty minutes, 50 percent NREM and 50 percent REM, shifting through three to four hours. A lot of mothers have experienced that infants do not always sleep nice and smoothly, but that is because of many different reasons not described in this book. However, I think that you can see signs of bad sleeping quality in very young children, not from any diseases, but just inherited weaknesses from the family tree.

Kevin Nelson and associates from the University of Kentucky in Lexington found that people who report having a near-death experience are more prone to also have experienced blurring of their awake and sleep states. This medical condition is known as REM intrusion. Sixty percent of those who reported having had near-death experiences also reported at least one occurrence of their REM sleep state intruding into their awake state, compared with only 24 percent of those without near-death experiences.

One explanation for decreased performance in sleep deprivation is the occurrence of microsleep. Microsleep is defined as brief (several seconds) runs of theta or delta activities that break through the otherwise beta or alpha EEG of waking. It has been seen to increase with sleep deprivation. In studies in which polysomnography is recorded simultaneously, microsleep impairs continuity of cognitive function and occurs prior to performance failure. One guess would be that microsleep occurs sadly in motor accidents due to sleep deprivation. Sometimes you get away with it, but unfortunately not all the time.

Dream State

After years of science, there is still much mystery about how the brain works during sleep. Ullrich Wagner, a researcher from Germany, found that the brain interprets and restructures information received during the day. He suggested that our brains determine solutions to complex problems during sleep, which we realize only after we awake. You must have read that many times, scientists have awakened and suddenly had solutions to a tricky problem. Often the answer to a problem is simpler than you expected at the beginning. So the phrase "let me sleep on it" is more true according to science than most people believe. It is amazing how very real a dream can be, almost like being awake; I have been thinking this many times during the years. Is this just a dream or a second reality? We can't be without a dream phase, our "twin" reality. According to my knowledge, all theories about why we dream are just speculations; nobody really knows for sure.

Through REM sleep, you get access to your dream state, although there are some dreaming phases in NREM. There have been uncountable numbers of books written about dreams, countless interpretations of dream scenarios and how the dream play interacts with our daily life. But are there any proofs about the essence of dreaming? I'm not sure myself. Most of the theories say that it's about humans' or mammals' brains having ways to collaborate with our daily life. The question is this: Are there any changes in life when following your dreams?

Although I admit it's a very interesting field to dig into and to investigate, more answers about dreams have yet to come. I'm just amazed how real a dream can be; it must be there for a purpose. I used to think, "A dream can be so real that you can almost touch it." And it's amazing how complicated dream scenarios can be. Consider that our physical world consists of four dimensions (length, width, height, and time), but the dream state doesn't need all those dimensions to be real. It's like all dimensions are just thrown into our brain, and it becomes so vivid and real. If you can dream it, you can live it. Perhaps that is the reason that dreams are so important.

One of my more frequent dreams (to tell a nice one) is my ability to fly, which would be one of humans' ultimate wishes in real life. The interpretation; if you fly with lot of joyfulness and with little effort, it means you have everything under control at your helicopter site. I must admit, this dream seems to come more frequently in certain periods, which may mirror my life situations at that time.

What about nightmares? Everybody has those unpleasant dream events, when you wake up bathed in sweat. How do you interpret a dream when your heart is beating? However, I had a special nightmare starting as a child and continue many years, it didn't fad a way until a grown up person. But it took me many years to explain or to interpret my dream. My mum used to ask me what the dream was about, but I could never say, it just scared me. But in my late twenties it struck me, suddenly. My dream was a memory from my past and not just a regular dream scenario. I got a glimpse before my birth. It was not about anything, just a sequence inside my mum's whom and the feeling I had at that moment. As one child of two, twins, it was pretty crowed and we had to leave the accommodation rather hasty (me, 12 min before my brother) two months before the normal schedule. I suppose, it was a rough time for me and therefore had an impact later in my life. If I had known the truth from the beginning it would had helped me and not scared me, as it did.

Experts say that one reason for nightmares may be a way for your unconscious to get your attention about a situation or problem you have been avoiding. Sometimes nightmares serve to warn you about your health or an accident. I have just one question mark. We can't remember most of our dreams, so how are we getting any help from them? Perhaps it may be from our subconscious. Questions? Yes! Answers?-No! Anyway, discussing, analyzing, and understanding your nightmares can lead to a solution for your problem, they say. As I mentioned before, there are many solutions in trying to understand the meaning of dreams. Some more answers:

Sigmund Freud, the father of psychoanalysis (1856–1939), suggested that bad dreams let the brain learn to gain control over emotions resulting from distressing experiences. He believed that nothing occurs by chance, that every action and thought is motivated by your unconscious. He revolutionized the study of dreams with his work *The Interpretation of Dreams*.

Carl Gustav Jung (1875–1960), like his mentor Freud, also believed in the existence of the unconscious, but he saw it in a more spiritual way. He suggested that dreams may compensate for one-sided attitudes held in waking consciousness. The dreams are guiding you to achieve wholeness.

Antti Revonsou, a Finnish professor and philosopher, suggested that dreams serve the purpose of allowing for the rehearsal of threatening scenarios in order to better prepare an individual for real-life threats. This theory rests on the widely accepted observation that most remembered dreams are stressful—filled with negative emotions and dramatic conflicts.

A more extensive view of "dreaming as play" was proposed by Nicholas Humphrey of the Centre for Philosophy of Natural and Social Science: we dream to practice many different physical, intellectual, and social skills, not just to resolve past threats.

Crick and Mitchison believe that "cortical neural networks become overloaded during learning and that the function of REM sleep is to remove superfluous connections by randomly flooding them." In an article in *Nature* in 1983, they wrote: "We propose that the function of dream sleep is to remove certain undesirable modes of interaction in networks of cells in the cerebral cortex, by a reverse learning mechanism, so that the trace in the brain of the unconscious dream is weakened, rather than strengthened, by the dream." Crick and Mitchison pointed out that almost all mammals and birds—animals that have a neocortex or similar structure—experience REM sleep. Psychoanalysis can't explain why even tiny moles experience REM sleep.

Joe Griffin and Ivan Tyrrell described what turns out to be a strikingly simple and satisfying explanation for why we dream and why the content of our dreams is so very often bizarre. They wanted to show that dreaming is vital for mental health (even though remembering dreams is not) and that the sleep state we associate with dreaming (the REM state) also has crucial importance when we are awake. That explains what we have known for a long time: depressed people sleep poorly, and bad sleep can cause depression. Still, we don't really know why we dream, what dreams mean, and how we can take advantage of them.

However, perhaps we will be better able to comprehend dreams in the future. New discoveries from a person's dream revealed "the first brain image created of a dream." The participant, a lucid dreamer, knew that he was dreaming and could control the scenes, said study coauthor Michael Czisch of the Max Planck Institute of Psychiatry in Munich, in an article in *Current Biology*. Monitoring the brain of a man who has unusual control over his dreaming made this research possible. By giving this participant instruction (by squeezing hands) during his lucid dream and then repeating the same instructions in a fully awake condition, Czisch showed there was boosted activity in similar brain regions, whether the hand squeezing was performed, imagined, or dreamed. I must say, many times I've been dreaming knowing that it was a dream and have been almost awake, but I couldn't do anything about it. Perhaps that is the strange thing about these results: to have control instead of being paralyzed.

Sleep in Adults

The world's aging population is increasing in numbers, which has a significant impact on society. Older people have different requirements from society and government as opposed to younger people. Older adults make up a large percentage of the population. Average life expectancy will increase at a rate of two years per decade, which means a growing aging population in the future. Therefore, age-related issues will have a big impact on every country and society. Sleep disturbances increase with aging.

According to NSF's 2003 sleep in America poll, 44 percent of older persons experience one or more nighttime symptoms of insomnia at least a few nights per week or more. If looking at Stages 3 and 4 changing with age, the percentages below speak for themselves. Men in the following age categories reported spending the following percentages of time in the SWS stage:

- Ages 20–29 years: 21 percent
- Ages 40–49 years: 8 percent
- Ages 60–69 years: 2 percent

From the above, you can see that elderly people's sleep has only a small amount of deep sleep. What can you expect from your sleep when you retire? If you compare the sleep you had in your younger years with when you were ending your career, only 10 percent of deep sleep is left when you pass sixty-five years of age. Older adults spend less time in the deeper levels of sleep, have more awakenings, and experience a reduction in REM sleep.

We know that old age means expected changes in sleep features. The declining time spent in slow-wave sleep (SWS) results in more time spent in the previous stages of sleep. REM sleep is generally preserved, but latency to the first REM period decreases, and the overall amount of REM sleep may decrease as a result of an overall reduction in nocturnal sleep time. Aging patients have a longer light sleep period, and they often experience reduced total sleep time and have more frequent awakenings.

Insomnia and *Stretch to Sleep*™-Program

Along with the physical changes that occur as we get older, changes to our sleep architecture are a part of the normal aging pattern. As people age, spend more time falling asleep, and have more trouble staying asleep, compared to when they were younger. Most older adults, though certainly not all, report being less satisfied with sleep and more tired during the day.

Decreasing:

- REM sleep
- Sleep efficiency
- Slow wave sleep

Increasing:

- Sleep latency
- Arousals/awaking
- Stage 1 and Stage 2

Studies on the sleeping habits of older Americans show an increase in the time it takes to fall asleep, an increase in sleep latency, and an overall decline in REM sleep. Also, an increasing sleep fragmentation occurs, which means waking up during the night. Some researchers (NSF) believe that it's a common misconception that sleep needs decline with age. They believe that our sleep can remain constant throughout adulthood. So what's keeping seniors awake? I believe that when seniors retire after a long life of working, it might be too abruptly. Maintaining a busy, interesting lifestyle, without your normal stress, can do the trick. Get up in the early morning and have a day of duties, which I know can be hard for some. Hobbies and social life can actually maintain sleep rhythm as an individual ages.

Changes in the patterns of our sleep, which specialists refer to as sleep architecture, may contribute to sleep problems. The sleep cycle is repeated several times during the night, although total sleep time tends to remain constant. Research on older patients has shown that they tend to fall asleep during the day faster than younger patients. The daytime sleepiness noted in this age group suggests that older adults may not be getting sufficient sleep at night, which may result from their disrupted ability to sleep. However, some researchers suggest that much of the sleep disturbance among the elderly can be attributed to physical and psychiatric illnesses and the medications used to treat them. That's not hard to digest. We have all seen in papers or have experience of older people with an arsenal of different medicines in their cupboards.

Women experience increased sleep disturbances as they age, which shows in the longer time to fall asleep and waking up more often at night; therefore, they are more tired during the day. Hot flashes and night sweats, associated with decreased levels of estrogen, may contribute to nightly awakenings. One of the golden rules of sleep is to make your body temperature fall; otherwise your body systems are not switched off. There are other factors affecting sleep during this period, including pain, certain medical and emotional conditions, and physical discomfort. Polysomnographic changes of elderly women's sleep have the same pattern as older persons overall, including decreased slow-wave sleep stages 3 and stage 4.

Circadian Rhythm

The circadian rhythm is roughly a twenty-four-hour cycle in the biochemical, physiological processes of living entities, including plants and animals among others. French scientists did premodern observations of the circadian oscillation in leaves back in 1700. But a great deal of research on biological clocks was done much later, in the second half of the 1950s. The term was first named in modern time by Franz Halberg, who worked at the University of Minnesota. The name *circadian rhythm* comes from Latin: *circa* means around, and *dies* means day. This literally translates as "rhythm around the clock." For some reason, it is just roughly twenty-four hours (24.2 hours). The reason why seems to be unclear to science, but the rhythm expands if you are exposed to a great deal of light in the evening or otherwise. Perhaps that's why it's essential to keep your rhythm in order; otherwise, it's easy for you to lengthen your rhythm ahead. Modern science nowadays tells us that a single cell has a circadian clock within it. At the same time, different cells may communicate with each other in synchronized ways.

The central clock that regulates the circadian cycles is located in two tiny structures in the brain, at the base of the left and right hypothalamus, and contains twenty thousand neurons. These structures are called the suprachiasmatic nuclei because they are located just above the optic chiasma, where the left and right optic nerves cross paths. The neurons of these nuclei use this information to resynchronize themselves with daylight every day, because like any clock, the human biological clock is not perfect and does need to be reset periodically.

More or less independent circadian rhythms are found in many organs and cells in the body outside the suprachiasmatic nuclei (SCN), the master clock. In mammals, the circadian system is hierarchical and responsible for regulating locomotors' activity rhythms and for synchronizing peripheral oscillators. These peripheral oscillators are found in the esophagus, lung, liver, pancreas, spleen, thymus, and skin.

Remember the saying "There is nothing new under the sun"? Old Oriental health theory determined long ago that human organs have their own specific clock or rhythm. This knowledge has now been reinvented in the Western world. For instance, in some hospitals in Germany, doctors treat cancer in accordance to the specific time to treat a particular organ. If you do just that, you can assure the highest benefits or response for the treatment and healing process to progress.

The suprachiasmatic nucleus sets the body clock to approximately 24.2 hours. A practical purpose has been proposed for the circadian rhythm using the analogy of the brain being somewhat like a battery charging during sleep and discharging during the awake period. A malfunction or mutations on the circadian clock gen, Clock Per-2, can lead to a delayed sleep phase. Circadian rhythms coordinate the timing of our bodily functions, including sleep. The sleep rhythm can be shifted forward so that seven or eight hours of sleep are still obtained, but the individuals will wake up extremely early because they have gone to sleep quite early. For example, older people tend to become sleepier in the early evening and wake earlier in the morning compared to younger adults. This pattern is called the advanced sleep phase syndrome. The reason for these changes in sleep and circadian rhythms as we age is not fully understood, but many researchers believe it may have to do with light exposure and a lack of outdoor light intake.

Exposure to light stimulates a nerve pathway from the retina in the eye to the suprachiasmatic nucleus, which initiates signals to other parts of the brain that control hormones, body temperature, and other functions that play a role in making us feel sleepy or wide awake. Treatment for advanced sleep phase syndrome normally includes bright light therapy. Another possibility for circadian rhythm changes involves changing the daily sleep schedule.

You will have a very rough experience with the offset of your circadian rhythm when travelling across a number of time zones. The body clock will be out of sync with the destination time, as it experiences daylight and darkness contrary to the rhythms to which it has grown accustomed. The body's natural pattern is upset, as the rhythms that dictate times for eating, sleeping, hormone regulation, and body temperature variations no longer correspond to the environment—nor to each other in some cases. To the degree that the body cannot immediately realign these rhythms, this condition is called jet lag.

Insomnia and *Stretch to Sleep*™-Program

To measure the circadian rhythm, you have classic phase markers:

- Body temperature
- Melatonin

Body Temperature

Body temperature cycles are under hypothalamic control. An increase in body temperature is seen during the course of the day and a decrease during the night. People who are alert late in the evening have body temperature peaks late in the evening, while those who find themselves most alert early in the morning have body temperature peaks early in the morning. The core body temperature of an individual tends to have the lowest value in the second half of the sleep cycle; the lowest point is one of the primary markers for circadian rhythms. The body temperature also changes when a person is hungry, sleepy, or cold.

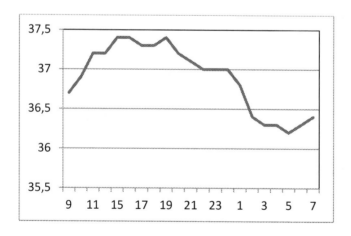

Figure 4. A human's body temperature during twenty-four hours

The average human adult's temperature reaches its minimum at about five o'clock in the morning, about two hours before the average waking time. Melatonin secretion starts at nine in the evening and ends at seven.

As everybody knows and experiences, good sleeper or not, body temperature doesn't follow that smooth, almost sinus-curve shape every night. An error in regular body temperature behavior is one of the reasons you wake up in the middle of the night bathed in sweat. In my experience, following the raised body temperature is demonstrated when you wake up finding it very easy to start thinking, looking at the day's issues, and trying to solve them. That's very right in a biological sense; your brain is warm too, like during daytime. It's easier to think when warm than when cold. Your brain slows down when body temperature declines.

In 1976, Horne and Ostberg found that morning types had higher daytime temperatures, with an earlier peak time than the evening types; also, they went to sleep and awoke earlier. Humans are normally diurnal animals, active in the daytime. Chronotypes are an attribute of human beings reflecting whether they are alert and prefer to be active early or late in the day. People are often referred to as "larks" and "owls," where morning people wake up early and are most alert in the first part of the day and evening people are most alert in the evening hours and prefer to go to bed late. Most people are neither evening nor morning types, but lie somewhere in between. Those people sharing the same type have similar activity patterns in terms of sleep, appetite, and exercise. Normal variation in the sleep/wake cycle is about two hours earlier or later. Going out from this range can cause problems in day-to-day life, normal work, and social activities.

Melatonin

Melatonin is a naturally occurring hormone found in animals and in some other living organisms, and is important in the regulation of the circadian rhythms of several biological functions. In higher animals, including humans, melatonin is produced by pinealocytes in the pineal gland and also by the retina, lens, gastrointestinal tract, and other tissues. The largest organ in humans to biosynthesize melatonin is the skin. These molecules are naturally synthesized from the amino acid tryptophan (via synthesis of serotonin). Serotonin is converted to melatonin by the enzymes N-acetyltransferase.

Melatonin is also a powerful antioxidant (discovered in 1993) and can easily cross cell membranes and the blood-brain barrier. In animals, melatonin has been demonstrated to prevent damage to DNA by some carcinogens, stopping the mechanism by which they cause cancer, although serum melatonin has a very short half-life (twenty minutes). The short half-life of melatonin is, of course, a negative factor for everybody with low serum melatonin production.

The suprachiasmatic nucleus (SCN), in the anterior hypothalamus, is thought to be the body's anatomic timekeeper, is stimulated from outside signals from the environment, and is responsible for the release of melatonin. The retina cells transmit, and integrate, light signals via the retionohypothalamic tract to stimulate the SCN. The SCN works like a clock that sets off a regulated pattern of activities that affect the entire body. During the day, the pineal is very low or inactive. Its onset in dim light, dim-light melatonin onset (DLMO), at about nine o'clock in the evening can be measured in the blood or in the saliva.

However, newer research indicates that the melatonin offset may be the most reliable marker. Benloucif and associates in Chicago in 2005 found that melatonin phase markers were more stable and more highly correlated with the timing of sleep than the core temperature minimum.

Melatonin produced by the pineal gland is under the influence of the SCN of the hypothalamus, which receives information from the retina about the presence or lack of light. Once exposed to the first light each day, the clock in the SCN begins performing functions like raising the body temperature and releasing stimulating hormones like cortisol. Even if the pineal gland is switched "on" by the clock, it will not produce melatonin unless the person is in a dimly lit environment.

In addition to sunlight, artificial indoor lighting can be bright enough to prevent the release of melatonin. That's one reason why modern life has a negative impact on sleep regulation in human. Even so, many people these days want to have bright and light bedrooms, and if it's possible, with large windows. But the sleep quality is not the same in the summertime compared to the cooler periods of the year. Normally, heat and light are enemies to good sleep.

It is very common and popular these days to take tablets of melatonin. There is not always an easy way, however, for melatonin to be helpful. The correct dosage, method, and time of day it is taken must be taken under consideration for the sleep problem. Taking it at the wrong time of the day may reset your biological clock and give you an unexpected reaction. For some people, melatonin seems to help improve sleep. Overall, research indicates that sleep improved when melatonin was taken at the appropriate time for jet lag and shift work. The sleep drug Ramelteon acts specifically at the MT1 and MT2 receptors to promote sleep. In Sweden, Circadin (2mg) is a product for sale for use for a short time for insomnia to patients from fifty-five years of age.

When melatonin was given to people near their normal sleep time, the results differed from one study to the next. When given during the day, it promoted drowsiness and shortened sleep onset. Melatonin might help shift workers on irregular shifts who need to adjust their schedules. When taken in low doses at the appropriate time, melatonin can help advance or delay the sleep-wake cycle.

Melatonin's antioxidant activity may increase longevity; it has been shown to increase the average life span of mice by 20 percent in some studies. Melatonin interacts with the immune system, and in preclinical studies, melatonin may enhance cytokine production. Some studies also suggest that melatonin might be useful in fighting infectious disease. This means that if you are blessed with good sleep, it's an overall benefit for your health. Many studies have proclaimed that people with bad sleep have a weakened immune system. Is it bad sleep since birth or a weak system from an early age, or could it be both? Probably, which I am going to explain later, the whole issue is a matter of inherited weakness from family trees. You got it from your mother or father and have to do the best you can to bridge the gap.

A systematic review of clinical trials (Mills et. al) involving a total of 643 cancer patients using melatonin found a reduced incidence of death. Reduced melatonin production has been proposed as a likely factor in the significantly higher cancer rates in night workers. Melatonin has important chronobiological effects, including sleep-promoting actions, which are mediated through specific receptors located in the major circadian pacemaker, the suprachiasmatic nucleus (SCN). Melatonin has been used successfully in the treatment of insomnia in older individuals in circadian rhythm sleep disorder. Studies of the effects of melatonin on decreasing sleep latency and on total sleep have not always produced consistent results.

A reduction in sleep onset latency can be interpreted in various ways. In the case of melatonin, some investigators have implicated hypothermia in this process, although hypothermia, in addition to circadian phasing of the core body temperature, is only seen at high, pharmacological doses. It is still unknown whether Ramelteon induces hypothermia.

Jet Lag

Jet lag, medically referred to as "desynchronizes," physiological in nature, is a consequence of the alterations of the circadian rhythm. The condition is not linked to the length of flight, but to the east-west meridian distance travelled. A ten-hour flight from Europe to South Africa does not cause jet lag, since it is a flight from north to south. On the other hand, a five-hour flight from the East to the West Coast of the United States may well result in jet lag. The condition of jet lag may last many days, and recovery rates of one day per eastward time zone or one day per one and half westward time zones. The speed at which the body adjusts to the new schedule depends on the individual; some people may require several days to adjust to a new time zone, while others experience little disruption. Crossing one or two time zones does not typically cause jet lag. When travelling across time zones, we need to adjust our body clocks from home time to the new time. The more time zones that are crossed, the longer it takes to reset the body clock to the new time. British Airways takes the problem seriously and provides a "jet lag calculator" for potential customers.

One study found that about half of all business travelers experience jet lag. They report that their performance and productivity are negatively affected; the problem was worse for women than men. There is no best cure for jet lag. You can use the power of the sun (or other sources of bright light) to reset your body clock. As a general principle, light exposure in the morning will reset the body clock to an earlier time, while light in the evening will reset it to a later time.

Since the experience of jet lag varies among individuals, it is difficult to assess the efficacy of any single remedy. However, there is research that gives us hope in this matter. A study by researcher Professor Andrew Loudon of Manchester University stated: "We've discovered that we can control one of the key molecules involved in setting the speed at which the clock ticks and in doing so we can actually kick it into a new rhythm." The research focused on an enzyme called casein kinase, which helps fine-tune the biological clock. In an experiment on mice, the study showed the drug blocked the enzyme and restarting clocks that had stopped. The study is said to be the first to tackle the essence of the body clock terminology.

What about eating on an international flight with many hours spent in a cabin and very little space to walk about? The key issue is when you start your flight. Previous research suggested that travelling on an empty stomach could help beat jet lag. Following that theory, US researchers Saper and associates recommended not eating at all while in the air for rapidly adjusting to another time zone. From my own experience with long flights, a tummy full of food makes it hard to sleep. It's not a problem with day flight, but even a small portion of dinner can be devastating if served too late. However, the recommendation not to eat at all is not something I find disturbing.

Shift Work

Shift work is another occasion in your daily life when you can experience problems in the circadian rhythm. Humans are believed to function at their best during the day, so working shifts is not natural behavior for the human body, even though some people manage better than others. A shift worker is anyone who follows a work schedule that is outside of the typical nine-to-five business day, but you can also experience the same problems if you work many hours overtime. In the past few decades, the industrial countries (and soon the whole world) have become increasingly dependent upon shift workers to meet the demands of globalization and our twenty-four-hour society. We have become more and more used to having everything every time we want it, and shift work is one way to increase production and customer service without major increases in infrastructure.

New findings may help explain why shift workers, people with sleep disorders, and others who disrupt their circadian rhythms by staying up late or eating meals at the wrong time tend to be more vulnerable to heart disease. Recently, scientists have discovered that the liver and other organs have their own internal clocks that may work independently of the brain clock and are set by mealtimes or other cues. Broken biological clocks in blood vessels may contribute to hardened arteries, even if the main timer in the brain works fine. Scientists assumed that the diseases resulted from malfunctions in a master clock in the brain, which synchronizes sleeping, waking, and other body functions with the rising and setting of the sun. Scientists tested (Cheng et. al) the theory by putting arteries from mice with broken clocks into normal mice, which resulted in the walls of the transplanted arteries becoming thick and less flexible, indicating that diseases may result from timing defects in the vessels, not the brain or the rest of the body.

Sometimes shift work can be a good solution for many families, to help to put together the daily schedule. There are millions of people who are considered shift workers, including doctors and nurses, pilots, builders, policemen, customer service representatives, commercial drivers, and so on. However, while shift work does create productivity, at the same time, it can result in seriously bad output. In the past, there have been many catastrophes with thousands of dead, that can be blamed on sleepiness and fatigue at work. Two of the most serious and persistent problems shift workers face are frequent sleep disturbance and associated excessive sleepiness. Those conditions can lead almost every time to poor concentration and absenteeism.

Consider that shift workers are often employed in the most dangerous of jobs, such as firefighting and emergency medical services. I have thought of that issue occasionally, since my brother Peter has worked many years on the police force in Stockholm, and sometime not slept properly. When these people need all the concentration they can get, their body has low biochemical storage of everything.

What can be done is to improve overall sleep for everybody, despite all the problems that come with shift work. Improving sleep will in the end have a big impact on productivity, health, and social interaction. In fact, to ignore the needs of the shift worker is only to look for short-term benefits and not try to find a better solution for generations to come. You could say that not everybody is made to deal with bodily excesses, or that some bodies are very sensitive to outside stimuli. According to the International Classifications of Sleep Disorder, people who suffer from sleep disturbances and excessive sleepiness in trying to adapt to a shift-work schedule are at increased risk for different types of chronic illnesses, such as cardiovascular and gastrointestinal diseases.

Power Nap

The expression *power-nap* was coined by Cornell University social psychologist James Maas. This is an expression used frequently in the last decade, and the essence is to rest your body and mind without coming into a deep sleep state, like state 2. By taking a power nap, you can gain energy quickly, in a short period of time. In Sweden, a famous former wrestler Martin Lidberg, a gold medalist in the European and world championships, practiced this technique many times, often before he started a hard exercise session. He said, "I don't sleep more than twenty minutes, and in the same time, gain two hours of waking time."

There are occasions when you need to power nap, for instance, in a spaceship in an orbit around earth. A NASA study by Graeber and associates examining the effects of a forty-minute rest period on the flight decks of commercial airliners showed that, during actual operations, a brief nap can significantly increase performance and alertness. The duration of the nap should be limited to about forty-five minutes or less; however, this is no substitute for actual sleep. Crew members are likely to feel most sleepy between 2:00 a.m. to 8:00 a.m. and from 2:00 p.m. to 5:00 p.m., and therefore these occasions are particularly good times to take advantage of this naturally occurring sleep tendency by napping.

I talked to a friend who exercised in a fitness center where I work. He always trained after work and very late in the evening. I asked him if he could sleep after a hard training session.

"No, I usually go to bed at two o'clock in the night and then go up at six in the morning," he said.

"How can you still have power left to train in the evening?" I replied.

"Well, I take a nap when I come home from work. I usually sleep for one and a half hours."

That explained the whole picture. For most people it's hard to sleep when training excessively. One and a half hours is often too much sleep to be considered a nap.

My friend had a hard time trying to balance late training with good sleep in too few sleeping hours. He was tired when he came home and had to restore energy to build muscles. I think he would gain a lot by just napping for twenty to thirty minutes; more than that can interfere with your regular sleep habit and rhythm. Longer naps can make it more difficult to fall asleep at night, especially if your sleep deficit is relatively small. Research has shown that a one-hour nap has many more restorative effects than a thirty-minute nap, including a much greater improvement in cognitive functioning. But if your naps interfere with your night sleep, you gain nothing.

Sleep Hygiene

Many researchers believe that there is a link between behavior and insomnia; therefore, behavioral therapy is often part of the treatment for insomnia. For example, bedtime routines or the bedroom itself may become linked with anxiety for a person who is experiencing insomnia. A combination of several behavioral treatments is typically the most effective approach, doctors say. Behavioral therapy alone is normally not enough; it would be too easy. In insomnia theory, behavioral therapists or doctors use the words "sleep hygiene" as key words for behavior and environmental factors, as they play a vital role in promoting sleep.

Develop Regular Sleep Habits

Try to go to bed at the same time every evening. Keep a regular schedule and develop regular habits before going to bed. Every person has the best time, or moment, in the evening for when he or she goes to bed. Don't do things you know are bad for your sleep. Don't do projects that will take too much mental energy from you. It is easy to start a home project for the evening, but it's harder to stop in time. Therefore, stimulating activities should be avoided an hour before bedtime; that includes tense activity like movies, television, and novels. This is very good advice and could be crucial, because for a good sleeper, a movie is like a sleeping pill, but for people with insomnia problems, it's just the opposite. For them, a movie is like a trigger for the arousal system. A sleeper can easily stop watching (or just fall asleep) in the middle of the movie and go to bed, but for a non-sleeper, this is nearly impossible—he or she has to see the end. For some of us, a tense movie is not what our body needs before going to bed. You cannot neglect the fact that the more activities you add in the evening, the harder it will be to relax.

Reserve the Bedroom Only for Sleeping

People should use their beds and bedrooms only for sleep and sex, doctors used to say. But a lot of people want to end a difficult day by reading their favorite book (like my brother). This habit can be good or bad; it depends. If you don't have any problems with reading at night, everything is fine. On the other hand, if you read and then can't sleep, you should change your routine. As I mentioned before, you must be aware of your routine and the arousal level it causes.

Environmental Triggers

Environmental triggers can include noise or trouble in your near surroundings. Being too hot or too cold can keep you awake. In the summertime, everyone has experienced sweaty nights without any good sleep. Sometimes it can be the opposite. I think everybody knows couples, if not themselves, who have different air needs or temperature needs. Some are draft susceptible, while others love open windows all night, every night. This is a tricky situation when the members of a couple have different needs. Sometimes love and sleep don't go hand in hand.

Food Restrictions

As you already know, food can cause bad sleep, but oftentimes it's the first pick for people who are anxious at night. Avoid large meals near bedtime. A full belly in the night does not improve your sleep. One main aim for better sleep is to reduce the body temperature. It has been shown in animal trials that animals that ate less but slept more lived longer, compared to animals that ate as much as they wanted but slept less. That is exactly how you find the Western world today; the scenario is similar. Among populations in several countries, mostly in the United States and United Kingdom, the picture is very clear and the same. There is a lot of stress, wrong eating habits, fewer sleeping hours, and bad quality of sleep. Many health care institutions in many countries recommended cutting down fat, which ended up in insulin resistance. People started to eat too much carbohydrate (pasta, potatoes, and bread). A strong sleeper doesn't mind a lot of food or stress; he or she just sleeps. But for others, mind your habits; they will interrupt your nights in a bad manner. To be totally frank, my feeling is that if you sleep well, whatever you do, it might get you in the end. If you look at the constitution patterns, good sleepers are slower and don't move and exercise enough, so they might be at higher risk to suffer high blood pressure and become overweight.

Consumption of tryptophan-containing foods may help induce sleep. Amino acids, including tryptophan, act as building blocks in protein biosynthesis. In addition, tryptophan functions as a biochemical precursor for the following compounds: serotonin (a neurotransmitter), synthesized via tryptophan hydroxylase. Serotonin, in turn, can be converted to melatonin. Tryptophan is a routine constituent of most protein-based foods or dietary proteins. It is particularly plentiful in chocolate, oats, durians, mangoes, dried dates, milk, yogurt, cottage cheese, red meat, eggs, fish, poultry, sesame, chickpeas, sunflower seeds, pumpkin seeds, spirulina, and peanuts. Clinical research has shown mixed results with respect to tryptophan's effectiveness as a sleep aid, especially in normal patients. Tryptophan has shown some effectiveness for treatment of a variety of other conditions typically associated with low serotonin levels in the brain, such as seasonal affective disorder.

Avoid Stimulants

Avoid stimulants like caffeine for at least three or four hours before bed. Some people can drink caffeine during the evening, but that is mostly impossible for people with sleeping problems. Avoid caffeinated beverages in the late afternoon or evening because the stimulant activity of adenosine antagonism can promote hyperarousal. Avoid alcohol in the evening since this can worsen sleep disorders and lead to frequent arousals. While a small amount of alcohol promotes sleep (because it is relaxing) early in the night, more alcohol can lead to sleep disruption later in the night due to alcohol's disruption of melatonin storage.

Exercise

Exercise can be beneficial if it is not too late in the day. Insomnia patients do not find relaxing on the agenda as a natural phase of the day. Exercise is good for sleep because it can help the body to relax. Relaxing is something you have to learn to do;

you have to think about it as a regular duty. Exercise done early in the day can also be helpful in reducing stress and promoting deeper sleep, because when you are in good shape, your body system functions in a higher state. Exercise in the late afternoon or early evening can promote sleep, but heavy physical training in the late evenings normally worsens sleep problems for insomnia patients.

Light Therapy

For a circadian rhythm disorder, light-phase shift therapy is useful for sleep disturbances associated with circadian rhythm abnormalities. Patients may be exposed to bright light from either a light box or natural sunlight to help normalize the schedule. Light therapy has been in use to treat light depressive symptoms, as well as insomnia.

State of Misperception

According to doctors, there are patients with insomnia who have some degree of sleep-state misperception. To be sure about your sleeping pattern, it can be monitored and documented by a polysomnogram. A polysomnogram may be useful in determining the etiology of the sleep disturbance. Such studies may be helpful in determining sleep and wakefulness in the intensive care unit or the sleep laboratory.

Keep Bedroom Dark

Use blackout curtains. Avoid turning on the lights if getting up in the night; it may help to avoid a disruption in melatonin production. If you can't feel your way around in the dark, the next best thing is to use a small night-light. Living in a townhouse with streetlights banging at your window makes it difficult to block out the incoming light. Quality dark curtains do the trick. To have early morning light from a nice sun is not what you need when have many hours still to sleep before the morning alarm clock rings. You can frequently see these days, in a number of TV-programs, that there seems to be a trend to build grand bedroom windows. To wake up to early sunlight with astonishing scenery seems to be number one on the wanted list. During the wintertime, it's no problem at all, obviously, since the sun is sleeping too. Surely waking up earlier than needed can't be something that we should urge. Why? Those people planning for big bedroom windows must be good sleepers! I can't find any other answer to it. Keep the light out of your bedroom!

Warm Color in Bedroom

My experience and science say that dark green walls around us are what we need to sleep best and deepest. Don't listen to or look at the latest trend. Nowadays, everything is bathed in bright light and white colors. Only ten years ago, hospital regulations in Sweden said walls and ceilings must be painted white. I suppose this was for sanitary reasons, because it looks cleaner. Now the establishment says that color is good for human health and mood. They started to paint hospital walls with warm colors. What happened then? Suddenly people did the opposite; every apartment was painted white. It's now high fashion in the Western world to live in a gallerylike environment. No contrast, everything looking the same, and even most furniture and the kitchen are in white. It's not for me! Perhaps I'm conservative and can't adapt to new things. But not long ago, people used to paint everything white and buy white furniture when they retired; it was a sign of getting old. Avoid white in the bedroom!

Keep the Bedroom Cool

Seventeen degrees Celsius is a good temperature to sleep in. People with poor sleep are sensitive to hot environments. It's not very uncommon to see married couples with different temperature needs. The best state is when you have a freezing feeling when entering your bed and it will take some time to warm it up. That is the ultimate temperature for most sleepers. During that time, the body is lowering its overall temperature, which is important to enter the sleep state. The low temperature reduces overall body temperature, and then the right temperature occurs for a perfect sleep match. You have surely experienced during the summertime how it can be hard to go to sleep or stay in a sleeping state because of a too-hot bedroom.

Limit Liquids at Bedtime

Avoid running to the bathroom several times during the night. The body needs liquids, but not right before going to bed. Frequent running to toilets is a bad habit for people with sleeping problems. Perhaps a nice cup of tea is enough when going to bed. Alcoholic beverages are absolutely devastating for sleep qualities in most aspects. In a very small amount, it can calm your mood. But remember, alcohol destroys melatonin production. However, you can find melatonin in grapes. That's why it's better to drink wine than beer to prevent insomnia. Don't drink too much, though, before going to bed!

Use Stimulants in the Morning

This is a little bit controversial; some people say you should avoid all stimuli. That is correct. But to alert your body in the morning, to start the clock, it is wise to use stimuli. The faster you feel alert in the morning, the faster your body clock starts, and when the clock starts to tick earlier in the morning, the faster you feel tired in the evening.

Morning Exercise

The insomnia constitution is not made for hard work or heavy lifting. To keep in shape is good in many aspects of life—though as I have noted, training too late in the day is bad for sleep. This is a tricky question, because normally insomnia patients tend more toward stiff bodies. For that reason, it is better to train in the afternoon. For sleep quality, however, it is better to work out in the morning, to make sure to wake up the body and to start the clock. Oxygen is preferred when going to bed, but stiff muscles are not. Don't exercise too late!

Enough Space

This is a forgotten issue. You pick your man or woman for life. But you take sleep for granted. Love and good sleep don't have to go hand in hand. Sometimes you pick a person with a personality similar to yours. Do you have enough room to get rest? Everybody has surely experienced in their early years of first love, that there was no room needed then. But times change! The older you get, the more important your own space is. I surely want to stretch out in bed, and I get very irritable when it's not possible. Small things can have a big impact for everyone. The insomnia constitution is extremely influenced by incoming disturbances. It's easy to wake up, instead of continue sleeping, and sometimes the lack of space could have a negative influence that night.

I saw an episode on TV a couple years ago. It was a program where people with some idea stand in front of investors and beg for money. One time, a young married couple presented a business proposition—a divided bedsheet. There was a little string in the middle, just to show where to find the middle of the sheet. The couple had what they thought solved a problem. I want my space! Leave my space alone! To know your area, just touch the string, they thought. But they didn't get a lot of attention. In fact, the prominent millionaires said, "That is not useful; it can't be sold." I thought it was a good idea. When a couple claims their space, you have a line. It would be a modern form of the Maginot line, but in bed. But then I understood why the millionaires turned it down. They didn't understand the whole concept, probably because they all had very large and expensive beds at home.

Put Lower Body Parts High

Make sure that your feet are higher than your heart. If you have been feeling tiredness in your legs when coming home from work, it's even more important. This advice I can really recommend. Have you noticed, when putting up your legs when watching TV, for instance, you feel instantly relaxed and perhaps yawn? Why not try it in the bed? Even if you lie horizontally to start with, you can gain a lot to put your feet above your heart horizontal line and this will promote your nervous parasympathetic system even further. Gravitation promotes the yang activity, which means standing, sitting, walking, and so on.

Use Socks

Sometimes the floor draft makes your feet cold. Cold feet prevent sleep. A golden rule is this: warm feet and cold head, which we could extend to say: warm lower body and cold upper body. This will also lower your body temperature in general. Dr. Beata O'Donoghue (the London Clinic) explains: "Warm feet cause blood vessels to enlarge, dispersing heat and lowering your core temperature." I find socks very useful all year round. Well, it depends where you live, whether in a warm climate or a cold one. In summertime, wherever you live, it is more likely you need to cool your feet. Just don't get cold feet!

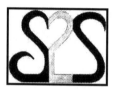

Part 2

Insomnia

Insomnia and *Stretch to Sleep*™-Program

Insomnia, which is Latin for *no sleep*, is the inability to fall asleep or remain asleep. Insomnia is also used to describe the condition of waking up and not feeling restored or refreshed, and it's also defined as a repeated difficulty with the initiation, duration, or quality of sleep that occurs despite adequate time. Sleep disorders are among the most common problems in medicine and psychiatry.

Studies (NIH Publ.) in the United States show that half of the population suffers more or less from poor sleep. An average American adult sleeps less than seven hours a night, compared to nine hours in 1910. In Sweden, a third of the population seems to have noticeable symptoms that can be related to sleeping problems. This proportion was only 12 percent at the start of 1990. So something has happened that has deteriorated sleep quality. The worldwide communications among people, faster each year, can bring a stressful life to us all. Having time for yourself is rare and getting harder to achieve each year. To be a good mother or father and at the same time have a career can be a daunting mountain to climb for most of us.

Sleep inability can result in very grave conditions and severe states of mind. Insomnia can be a diffuse disorder with significant social economic consequences, and it is a condition that is seen worldwide. One telephone survey in the United States showed nearly 33 percent of adults reported sleep disturbances.

Prognosis of sleep disturbance:

- US population 33%
- Europe and Japan population 22%

Two large epidemiological studies by Terzano and associates in Italy presented essential data on insomnia in patients whose primary provided health care was in Italy. The two insomnia studies clearly show that Italy has a high incidence of insomnia, which has a tremendous impact on health and public resources. The situation in Italy appears to be similar to other Western countries.

This syndrome has a great impact on mankind and is a considerable worldwide health issue, due to its influence on concomitant pathologies, increased burden on health-care resources, and the associated number of lost workdays. It is one of the most common clinical problems among the general population in every country, and especially in people with more complex conditions. Of course, everyone has experienced bad times in bed, with waking hours occasionally; for some reason or many reasons, we cannot sleep perfectly every night. But there are people who have almost no complaints at all. Still, one third of adults report some difficulty falling asleep or staying asleep during the past year, and 10 percent state the insomnia to be chronic or severe.

Whenever a patient reports unpleasant sleep despite an adequate duration of sleeping hours, doctors say the possibility of alterations in sleep related to pathologies or environmental aspects should be considered. It is important that information is collected on the daytime consequences of insomnia; patients often complain of tiredness, mood swings, reduced productivity, and anxiety about the upcoming night. If insomnia is creating serious effects, complicating other conditions, or making a person too tired to function normally during his or her waking hours, this would suggest that it is important to seek treatment. When effects are serious and untreated, insomnia can have a very bad impact on a person's health.

People with insomnia can experience the following:

- Excessive daytime sleepiness
- Difficulty concentrating
- Increased risk for accidents and illness
- Reduced quality of life

Insomnia of recent onset is often correlated with traumatic situations. While such insomnia may resolve spontaneously, it can also develop into chronic psychophysiological insomnia, in which acquired mechanisms strongly influence habitual sleep patterns. Science divides insomnia roughly into three different conditions: medical, psychological, and environmental. The severity of insomnia is related to the frequency of its manifestation, the number of nights per week during which the patient experiences sleep disturbance. Generally, insomnia can be considered severe when it presents at least three times per week.

Epidemiologic facts have shown that there is a greater risk for insomnia among the following:

Insomnia and *Stretch to Sleep*™-Program

- Women
- Elderly individuals
- People of lower socioeconomic status
- People with complex chronic conditions

According Sweden Statistics (SCB/ULF) there were 23 percent men and 35 percent women in the population who had difficulties with sleep. The huge difference between the start of this survey can be seen in 1986 when only 7 percent of the population aged 16-24 year have problem with sleep comparing to almost 24 percent 2007.

International Classification of Sleep Disorders

The International Classification of Sleep Disorders classifies insomnia into eleven categories, but for the purposes of this book, I have focused on just a few. The most interesting and severe states are those insomnia patients that have lifelong complaints and have gotten no help or results from treatment anywhere. I have described some of those categories below.

Acute Insomnia

Acute insomnia lasts less than three months. For example, insomnia due to a medical condition or mental disorder can have a quick impact or appear weeks before the emergence of the underlying mental disorder or medical reason. Insomnia due to drug or substance abuse can also have a fast impact.

Chronic Insomnia

Chronic insomnia means repeated difficulties with sleep initiation, maintenance, or quality of sleep and results in some form of daytime impairment. Chronic insomnia often begins as acute insomnia, which later develops into a chronic condition. Chronic insomnia is now accepted to occur in patients with predisposing or constitutional factors. Chronic insomnia can also develop from trigger factors, such as a major life event that brings the patient into an acute state of insomnia. If poor sleep habits or other constant factors occur in the following period of time, chronic insomnia occurs even if you remove the trigger. Chronic insomnia has numerous health consequences:

Reduced quality of life compared to other conditions such as:

- Diabetes
- Arthritis
- Heart disease

You can expect poor health, decreased activity, and an increased risk of mortality associated with short times of sleep.

Primary Insomnia

This sleeplessness is not from a medical, psychiatric, or environmental cause. Primary insomnia is more common in women than in men, with a female to male ratio of three to two. Hormonal variations may cause disruptions in sleep. Many other causes need to be excluded from the diagnosis of primary insomnia, for instance: chronic pain, especially neuropathic pain, and drug use or withdrawal. This type of insomnia, often termed "learned" insomnia, is more frequent in younger individuals.

Idiopathic Insomnia

This is where there is a longstanding complaint of insomnia, but the cause is not clarified. Lifelong sleeplessness is attributed to an abnormality in the neurological control of the sleep-wake cycle, typically beginning in early childhood. Insomnia tends to continue over the entire life span and can easily be aggravated by stress or tension. These individuals often show abnormal reactions, such as hypersensitivity or insensitivity to medications.

Primary and idiopathic insomnia are two different rubrics on nearly the same complaint. For me, it is not important to separate these two. The main question is this: Do you have trouble sleeping over a long time and for no reason at all? You feel that you have gotten no help anywhere. You are in the same boat as many other brothers and sisters worldwide, and it must be a pattern. I think there is something you can do about it.

Stimulants

Many people will connect to this section. This is about the daily or weekly stimulants used worldwide. "I have been drinking coffee, I have had a few drinks, and I have inhaled smoke (but only for a week)." Morning coffee is sometime, something you think about when going to bed in the evening. During one period of time, I changed from coffee to tea for six years, but nowadays I drink coffee regularly. It's very much a social thing, but it's also for achieving stimuli. How do stimulants interact with the human body? What can we expect of their impact on sleep quality? What is bad? What is good?

Stimulants are substances that induce a number of characteristic symptoms. Many users experience insomnia and anorexia, and some may develop psychotic symptoms. Stimulants have peripheral cardiovascular activity, elevating blood pressure and increasing the heart rate. Elevated mood, increased alertness, increased energy, insomnia, and anorexia are all common symptoms associated with stimulant use.

Long-term stimulant use may result in weight loss, as well as potential adverse psychiatric symptoms such as the following:

- Irritability
- Aggression
- Impulsivity
- Hallucinations
- Delusions

During stimulant withdrawal, you can experience a lot of unwanted effects, which are similar to or even more severe than the original effects of the stimulants. The most common stimulants in use are coffee, alcohol, and smoking.

Insomnia and Coffee

I knew early on that I couldn't drink coffee late in the evening if I expected a good night's sleep, but is coffee only bad for your sleep (for some people) or does coffee have a beneficial side as well? In recent years, it has become increasingly clear that coffee is more than just a morning routine. The body of data suggests that it can be beneficial for mental and medical conditions.

Coffee is one of the most popular beverages worldwide, and it is the world's most widely used central nervous system stimulant, with approximately 80 percent of the world's population being coffee consumers. Coffee was first consumed in the ninth century, when it was discovered in the highlands of Ethiopia. From there, it spread to Egypt and Yemen. The English word *coffee* first came to be used in the early to mid-1600. By the fifteenth century, coffee had reached northern Africa. It then spread to Italy, and then to the rest of Europe and on to Indonesia. Coffee has played an important role in many societies throughout modern history. Coffee is important for the export trade. In 2004, coffee was the top agricultural export for twelve countries (FAQ Yearbook); and in 2005, it was the world's seventh largest legal agricultural export by value.

Many studies have examined the relationship between coffee consumption and certain medical conditions; whether the overall effects of coffee are positive or negative is still in dispute. A coin has two sides, and drinking coffee seems to be equally divided in the good or the bad, speaking in the sense of biological advantage for humans. In a recent study by Freedman and associates (2012), a follow-up between 1995 and 2008, but in age-adjusted models, the risk of death was increased among coffee drinkers. However, coffee drinkers were also more likely to smoke, and after adjustment for tobacco-smoking status and other potential confounders, there was a significant inverse association between coffee consumption and mortality. Perhaps drinking coffee is not that bad for overall health, but if you are on the borderline of insomnia, it could be devastating. In other words, coffee may be good for your health but not for your sleep. On the other hand, using coffee in the right way can help you.

In adults, caffeine can affect arousal attention, reaction time, and sleep. Adults and many youth use caffeine daily, and caffeine use is associated with poor sleep and daytime fatigue. Understanding caffeine's effects on sleep is particularly important in clinical disorders such as depression, in which sleep difficulties are important features. Most people use it after waking up in the morning or to remain alert during the day. While it is important to note that caffeine cannot replace sleep, it can temporarily make us feel more alert by blocking sleep-inducing chemicals in the brain and increasing adrenaline production. It's a balancing act between the good and the bad when drinking coffee. When you wake up in the morning, it's important to be alert and to start the clock for the next sleep cycle, and caffeine does just that. However, insomnia may be exacerbated by stimulants, such as coffee, which disturb sleep continuity, leading to arousals and increased sleep latency. Be aware of the borderline, and don't over stimulate your arousal system.

Caffeine use may have an important association with sleep quality. There is evidence that, like adults, youth use caffeine to counteract daytime sleepiness. Caffeine use in youth tends to increase at the end of the week, after Wednesday. Epidemiological work (Morgan et.al) showed that caffeine use in youth was 75 to 98 percent, with at least one caffeinated beverage daily. The subjective effects of high caffeine doses on youth are similar to those found in adults, such as nervousness and nausea

There are numerous studies to support the idea that caffeine causes physical dependence. If you get a headache after not drinking your regular cups of coffee, your body is dependent on caffeine, and that it is something to think about. I for instance, "broke up" with caffeine for seven years. During that period of time, I felt I improved in every aspect of life, physical and mental, but I got bored just drinking tea. Also, I felt a little bit odd and antisocial as well.

Caffeine also increases the turnover of many neurotransmitters, including monoamines and acetylcholine. Adenosine decreases the neuronal firing rate and inhibits both synaptic transmission and the release of most neurotransmitters.

Youth with MDD (major depressive disorder) report (Whalen et al.) greater caffeine use and subjective sleep problems than healthy youth. Caffeine use is associated with greater sleep problems that night and greater negative effects that day, especially for youth with MDD. Contrary to what the researchers believed, caffeine use and sleep were not directly related to each other. They found that youth who used more caffeine did not report more trouble sleeping that night, with the exception of more awakenings at night. That was probably because coffee makes you go to the toilet more often, and therefore coffee drinkers had more awakenings during the night.

The risk for depression may decrease as coffee consumption increases, new research from 2011 (Lucas) suggests. In a ten-year cohort study of more than fifty thousand older women, investigators found that compared with those who drank one cup or less of caffeinated coffee per week, those who drank two to three cups per day had a 15 percent decreased risk for depression, and those who drank four cups or more had a 20 percent decreased risk. However, a study from Finland (Tanskanen et al.) found that although the risk for suicide decreased progressively for those consuming up to seven cups of coffee per day, the risk started increasing when consumption went over eight cups a day, We know that caffeine has an impact on the brain and on serotonin, which has been associated with depression.

A study published by the American Physiological Society (Bethesda) and based on research Australia found that glucose and insulin levels are higher with caffeine ingestion and stated the following:

- Four hours after exercise, the drink containing caffeine resulted in 66 percent higher glycogen levels compared to the carbohydrate-only drink.
- Several signaling proteins believed to play a role in glucose transport into the muscle were elevated to a greater extent after the athletes ingested the carbohydrate-plus-caffeine drink, compared to the carbohydrate-only drink.

The researcher explained that caffeine may increase the activity of several signaling enzymes that have roles in muscle glucose uptake during and after exercise. This finding might have a deeper impact on our society than we think. The Western world is drinking more and more coffee each year. Coffee machines for private consumption or those fast-spreading coffee shops everywhere provide us with café late or espresso whenever we want. Sometimes you want to hold back your sugar intake and therefore drink a straight one. Well, the research says that you increase your insulin level just by drinking a plain cup of coffee, and if you grab a biscuit as well, you might double dose.

A current study examined relationships between caffeine use and sleep in healthy and depressed youth. People who drink more than four caffeinated beverages a day are more likely to have difficulty falling asleep and wake unrefreshed. Most coffee drinkers have learned through the years how much they can drink before losing sleeping qualities. If you are in the category of moderate caffeine intake, you are probably not in any danger. Three cups of coffee per day is considered a moderate amount of caffeine. Six or more cups of coffee per day is considered excessive intake of caffeine.

The good effects of coffee are as follows:

- Increased alertness
- Increased metabolic rate

The bad effects of coffee are as follows:

- Reduced fine-motor coordination
- Headaches and dizziness
- Anxiety and nervousness
- Irritability
- Rapid heartbeat
- Excessive urination
- Sleep disturbance

Insomnia and Alcohol

In Western cultures, there are social habits connected to alcohol. Pubs, for instance, are meeting places for stressed inhabitants after work. In Sweden, we never had the same relationship as on the continent, although, the term "alcoholism" was first used in 1849 by the Swedish physician Magnus Huss to describe the systematic adverse effects of alcohol.

You can't buy spirits in a regular food store in Sweden, but that monopoly will maybe disappear in the future. Nowadays, there are restrictions against advertising alcohol brands. Alcohol kills, in the long run, science claims. In patients with alcoholic neuropathy, nutritional deficiency goes hand in hand with alcohol abuse. Harmful drinking is defined in the International Classification of Diseases (WHO)as a pattern of drinking that causes damage to physical (eg to the liver) or mental health (eg episodes of depression secondary to heavy consumption of alcohol).

Alcoholism is common, serious, and expensive. Physicians encounter alcohol-related diseases such as the following:

- Cirrhosis
- Cardiomyopathy
- Pancreatitis
- Gastrointestinal bleeding
- Intoxication

Alcohol concentrates more easily in the blood in older individuals, so the sedating effects are more powerful. Alcohol affects virtually every organ system in the body and, in high doses, can cause coma and death. It affects several neurotransmitter systems in the brain, including:

- GABA
- glutamate
- serotonin
- dopamine

Alcohol inhibits the receptor for glutamate. Long-term ingestion results in the synthesis of more glutamate receptors. When alcohol is withdrawn, the central nervous system experiences increased excitability. Persons who abuse alcohol over the long term are more prone to alcohol withdrawal syndrome than persons who have been drinking for only short periods. Alcoholism is slightly more common in lower income and less educated groups. Alcoholism is at least twice as prevalent in men as it is in women, although women are catching up. The lifetime prevalence was 20 percent in men and 8 percent in women. In Britain, one in three patients in community-based primary care practices had at-risk drinking behavior. In one year you can expect 1.64 million people to die from alcohol itself, and of course that number is far greater if you consider deaths related to alcohol.

The following apply to the US adult population from US National Longitudinal Alcohol Epidemiologic Study:

- Current drinkers 44 percent
- Former drinkers 22 percent
- Lifetime abstainers 34 percent

Women do not metabolize alcohol as efficiently as men. Hazardous drinking (not alcoholism) is greater than one drink daily for women and greater than two drinks daily for men. Binge drinking as a student can have devastating results, not only on your sleeping quality, but also on, for instance, breast cancer, even without any sign of breast cancer in the family. There are several cases of young women drinking to an alcoholic level in just a few years' time.

Although moderate drinking can offer health benefits, new research claims that abstinence following moderate drinking can lead to depression and weaken the growth of new neurons (neurogenesis) in the hippocampus. Summarizing her research study on mice, Jennie Stevenson stated that this is the first evidence that long-term abstinence from moderate alcohol drinking leads to negative mood state and depression.

Through the years, major catastrophes, man-made or natural, have had great impact on alcohol use. For instance, nine months after the attack on the World Trade Center, a survey found increased alcohol use was over 19 percent (Williams NIDA). The same pattern can be seen in combat veterans of the Gulf War.

What about sleep and alcohol? Well, most of us know by trial and error that a large dose of alcohol is devastating for sleep quality. You do get to sleep pretty fast, but you wake up after a while and then have difficulties getting back to sleep. That is mostly for one reason: alcohol makes melatonin deteriorate and vanish quickly from your body. But alcohol has a relaxing outcome in small doses, and therefore it is easy to use when coming home after work. As you know, this could be a deceiving strategy, though, in the long run.

Alcohol makes very specific marks on the sleeping architecture. Older patients may also have sleep disruption due to the use or abuse of alcohol, caffeine, and nicotine. Alcohol may be used by a significant proportion of those with insomnia, as it reduces sleep latency. Unfortunately, alcohol is notorious for producing sleep architectural fragmentations, like REM stage rebound or reduced sleep latency.

Moderate alcohol consumption thirty to sixty minutes before bedtime catalyzes disruptions in sleep maintenance and sleep architecture that are mediated by blood alcohol levels. Disruptions in sleep maintenance are most marked once alcohol has been completely metabolized from the body. In terms of sleep architecture, moderate doses of alcohol facilitate rebounds in rapid eye movement (REM) and stage 1 sleep; following suppression in REM and stage 1 sleep in the first half of an eight-hour sleep episode, REM and stage 1 sleep increase well beyond baseline in the second half.

My experience regarding sleep and alcohol is that you can choose between "bad" and "good" alcohol beverages, as well. Since I have been interested in and investigated sleep-related problems for many years, I firmly state that wine is preferred to beer for many reasons:

- Lower gluten
- Grape includes the melatonin hormone
- Less diuretic fluid

Insomnia and Smoking

My own experience of smoking is limited—only couple weeks, many years ago. I was away from school and secretly smoking with my brother and other schoolmates. That was "the adventure." For some reason, smoking wasn't for me or my brother and we stopped after a while. We managed throughout our lives without the influence of nicotine, and saved our lungs and cash.

But what about nicotine influences during the nighttime—what can we expect? Nicotine is an alkaloid found in the nightshade family of plants; it constitutes approximately 0.6 to 3.0 percent of the dry weight of tobacco, with biosynthesis taking place in the roots and accumulating in the leaves. In low concentrations (an average cigarette contains about 1 mg of absorbed nicotine), the substance acts as a stimulant in mammals, and it is one of the main factors responsible for the dependence-forming properties of tobacco smoking.

Cigarette smoking has numerous adverse effects on overall health, especially on the cardiovascular system, and smoking has been linked to total and cause-specific mortality in smokers. On average, 8.64 billion cigarettes are smoked each day of 1 billion users and 6.1 million deaths are caused by smoking each year. That is the size of the population of Norway. Male and female current smokers reported (Hannan et. al) less physical activity, greater consumption of alcohol and of red and processed meat, lower intake of fruits and vegetables and fiber, less multivitamin use, and a lower prevalence of colorectal endoscopy when compared with never smokers. The risk decreased with increased time since quitting and among former smokers who had quit before the age of forty or had abstained for more than thirty years.

Nicotine

As nicotine enters the body, it is distributed quickly through the bloodstream and can cross the blood-brain barrier. On average, it takes about seven seconds for the substance to reach the brain when inhaled. The half-life of nicotine in the body is around two hours, and it acts on the nicotinic acetylcholine receptors. In small concentrations, nicotine increases the activity of these receptors. A single amino-acid difference between brain and muscle acetylcholine receptors explains why nicotine activates the CNS but does not activate skeletal muscles and cause instant death. A cigarette stimulates the release of many chemicals. The release of neurotransmitters and hormones is responsible for most of nicotine's effects.

Nicotine appears to enhance the following key effects due to the increase of acetylcholine:

- Concentration
- Memory
- Alertness

Sleep and nicotine

A study was done in part of the larger Sleep Heart Health Study (2008), a multicenter study on sleep-disordered breathing and cardiovascular disease. The study subjects were matched with forty nonsmokers for age, sex, body-mass index, and race. There was no difference between smokers and nonsmokers in visual scoring, but the spectral analysis of brain-wave activity showed that compared with nonsmokers, smokers on average had a higher percentage of alpha power (15.6% vs. 12.5%) and a lower percentage of delta power (59.7% vs. 62.6%). This means that the smokers spent more time in light sleep and less time in deep sleep compared to nonsmoking counterparts. These are not very large percentage differences, but if you sleep at your margin, it could be a turning point. Many small negative activities can be devastating for your sleep quality.

Pharmacological Treatment

This book is not meant to be an encyclopedia of prescription drugs for your sleeping problems; it is actually the opposite. My hope is to give you other options besides drugs to deal with your sleep problems. Still, I want to give you a brief picture of how drugs work and stimulate the human systems to promote sleep.

It is obvious that prescribing drugs for sleeping problems is a delicate task, and everyone on both sides (doctors and patients) should be aware of "less is preferable." Unfortunately, I have had experiences with friends with habits of using sleeping pills for the relief of their night's terror. For some people, sleeping pills are the only solution, and they have no ending plans. They have difficulties in stopping the use of drugs, because their bodies are getting used to them.

I think most people have had some sort of relation to sleeping drugs for some period of time in their lives; even I did, but it was only for a very isolated time of use. My experience is that drugs can be used in times of reduced sleep for some reasons, but the body adapts very quickly to them. You should act if you don't need the full amount of sleep hours, because the system may have tuned in to another scale. To come back to your normal behavior, it might be necessary to take pills. That is the opposite strategy used for most sleep difficulties, when doctors sometimes use sleep-restriction programs. That means, when you already sleep too little, the prescription is to sleep even less.

Physicians have many different drugs for treating insomnia, but every situation is unique, and the complexity of the human body is like the number of the human's code of genes. For a pharmacological treatment to be effective, it should have sedative-hypnotic qualities, which means it will restore physiological sleep, both quality and quantity. Patient compliance is likely to be influenced by both the efficacy and the tolerability of the therapy.

As already mentioned, there is a complex relationship existing between insomnia and depressive disorders. It is not an easy task to be cured of depression if you still can't sleep at night. Treatment strategies should address both depressive symptoms and insomnia and should consider the use of both pharmacologic and no pharmacologic strategies, although most doctors believe that pharmacological treatment is the most practical approach to insomnia management because of its efficacy and its economic aspects. However, hypnotic drugs with a short half-life are preferable (the shorter the half-life, to the more preferable). Most of the time, hypnotic drugs are approved for two weeks or less of continuous use. But for chronic insomnia, longer courses may be indicated.

When using drugs, you hope for a rapid-acting effect and reduced sleep latency period. The drug should provide refreshing sleep, not only preventing nighttime awakenings but also restoring the number and duration of rapid eye movement (REM) and non-REM episodes to physiological levels. The drug should also be well tolerated, restore the patient's quality of life, and be easy for the patient to comply with treatment. Adverse events most commonly perceived by the patient include alterations in cognitive function, memory, and psychomotor activity, with negative effects on routine daily activities, of which the so-called hangover effect is a common manifestation. In addition, rebound insomnia can occur after abrupt withdrawal of hypnotic therapy.

BZDs were first introduced during the 1960s and quickly replaced barbiturates for the treatment of insomnia due to their broad therapeutic index. The efficacy of BZDs in patients with insomnia has been clearly demonstrated: they are highly effective at increasing duration of sleep and are characterized by a rapid onset of action. BZDs also tend to alter sleep patterns by increasing the activity of the sigma band (considered to be associated with protection against being awakened by external stimuli) and prolonging the duration of stage 2 sleep (a non-REM sleep phase). This can lead to a consequent reduction in REM sleep and a potential reduction in the quality of sleep. The use of BZDs has been associated with several collateral effects, which vary according to the specific agent, dosage, and half-life. These include hangover effects, loss of psychomotor performance, and rebound insomnia. Tolerance can also develop at high dosages.

Single Drug Intrusion

What can be expected as unpleasant effects from one single sleeping drug? Most of all, we are talking about serious negative outcomes in the long run, such as inflammation, enlargement, and restriction of organs. More specifically:

- Enlarged prostate
- Restricted urine tract, some part of stomach, duodenum
- Jaundice
- Mouth dryness
- Lack of eye liquid
- Increased reaction time
- Interaction with or against other drugs

I have noticed among friends that frequent use of sleeping drugs can have a devastating effect on your daily life. The above list includes several unwanted side effects, and even if an enlarged prostate is not malignant in any way, it can be a life-changing experience that can restrict your activities in practical living.

Categories of Drugs

- Benzodiazepines
- Hypnotic drugs
- Hormone replacement therapy
- Antidepressants
- Melatonin agonists

Benzodiazepines

Benzodiazepines are a group of drugs many of which have a strong sedative effect; they aim to help insomnia patients, with or without accompanying anxiety, producing drowsiness, and slowing down mental activity. In 1988, the United Kingdom's

Committee for Safety of Medicines (MHRA) issued guidance to GPs, advising that benzodiazepines should be prescribed for no more than two to four weeks, because of the high risk of addiction. Benzodiazepine prescriptions have fallen in the United Kingdom since their peak of 31 million a year in 1979, although there were still 10.7 million prescriptions for the drugs in 2008. But, still many reports publish about this drug. For instance, just in the very late of the completion of this book (Dec 2012) you could read about benzodiazepines is associated with an increased risk of developing and dying if pneumonia, according to a new study (published in Thorax online).

Benzodiazepines receptor agonists are used most frequently for insomnia. These drugs bind to a special benzodiazepine site on the GABA receptor complex. All have different metabolites that affect their onset and duration of action. These drugs have been the hypnotics of choice for many years because of their relative safety compared to barbiturates, which were the frequently used drug in the past. GABA is a chemical messenger that is widely distributed in the brain, and its natural function is to reduce the activity of the neurons to which it binds.

Intermediate- and long-action benzodiazepines are used for sleep-maintenance insomnia. When treatment is continued for more than thirty days, the hypnotic capacity of BZD drugs is clinically reduced. In the case of withdrawal, the drug should be gradually reduced in order to avoid rebound insomnia. Particular attention should be paid to use of BZD drugs in women and elderly patients, as their reduced hepatic metabolism can lead to amplification of the negative effects of BZD drugs, such as sedation and reduced attention span. As a consequence of residual sedative effects and accumulation of BZD drugs, for instance, memory and psychomotor performance can be affected. This reduction in daily psychomotor performance can lead to increased risk of a variety of accidents.

It is a short-acting drug, so it is a good agent for sleep-onset insomnia and has no significant residual effect in the morning. However, there is a high incidence of rebound insomnia and adverse effects, including dizziness, drowsiness, and headache. The drugs can depress CNS activity when administered with other drugs that interfere with CNS activity, but they reduce both the sleep latency period and the number of nighttime awakenings and increase the duration of sleep. Some drugs have no active metabolite, which reduces cognitive impairment and grogginess the following day.

Insomnia and *Stretch to Sleep*™-Program

Hypnotic Drugs

These non-benzodiazepine drugs are used for treatment of acute and short-term insomnia. Because of their sedative activity, this type of drug does not interfere with the physiological structure of sleep in healthy humans, and therefore they do not cause rebound insomnia or other related symptoms for durations that do not exceed a few weeks. The product consists of a coated two-layer tablet. The first layer releases drug content immediately to induce sleep; the second layer gradually releases additional drug to provide continuous sleep. The drug restores physiological sleep without compromising REM sleep. It also decreases sleep latency and increases duration of sleep.

Hormone Replacement Therapy

Estrogen replacement has been shown to improve sleep in menopausal women, primarily by reducing vasomotor symptoms that disturb sleep. In addition, it may improve sleep-related breathing disorders. Multiple aspects of menopause respond to estrogen replacement therapy. However, this has not been shown to be effective in treating depression associated with menopause. Frequent bad side effects include weight gain, edema, and breast tenderness.

Antidepressants

Antidepressants are indicated for use in patients with insomnia associated with psychiatric disorders or patients who have a previous history of substance abuse. Like other antidepressants, little scientific evidence supports their efficacy in the treatment of insomnia without associated depression.

Drug taking while still awake and active may cause hallucination, short-term memory impairment, impaired coordination, lightheadedness, and dizziness. The drugs are effective for treatment of clinical depression. Some are also indicated for panic disorders and obsessive, compulsive disorders. Intake with alcohol or other centrally acting drugs increases CNS depression.

Melatonin Agonists

The drug Ramelteon is indicated for insomnia characterized by difficulty with sleep onset and acts through melatonin receptor agonists, with high selectivity for human melatonin MT1 and MT2 receptors. MT1 and MT2 promote sleep and are involved in the maintenance of the circadian rhythm and normal sleep-wake cycle. Ramelteon is the first FDA-approved melatonin receptor agonist drug. Caution should be taken in mild hepatic impairment; adverse effects that led to discontinuation in clinical trials included dizziness, nausea, fatigue, headache, and worsening insomnia. The drug has also been associated with decreased testosterone levels and increased prolactin levels.

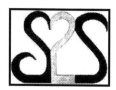

Part 3

S2S Program

in Theory

We already know from the previous chapter, for instance, from Dr. Ingaramo, that an abnormal activation of the sympathetic nervous system could damage blood vessels and vital organs. But long before that, a person is very likely to experience periods of bad sleep or insomnia—especially if you get an extra gear and overdrive the sympathetic nervous system and don't know how to pull the brake. As I describe later, some people have more of the "day system" and need to get more of the opposite system. The key task for all bad sleepers and an overall necessity for everyone is to know how to change their nervous system; therefore, here is just a brief explanation of the central nervous system, CNS.

For some reason, the number 100 billion appears frequently in nature. Scientists and astronomers often declare that our galaxy, the Milky Way, consists of just that number of stars, and that our galaxy is an average type in the universe, which consists of 100 billion galaxies. In the brain, the nervous system cells gather together in the same 100 billion number, but in tiny neurons. The neurons work out electrochemical impulses from everywhere in the body, and after these signals have been interpreted, they are sent back to various glands and muscles. Nerve cells have two types of body, called dendrites and axon.

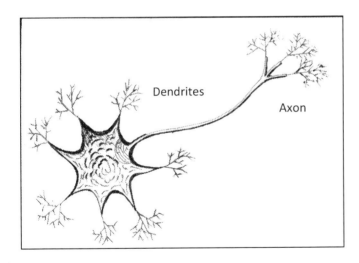

Figure 5. Two-dimensional nerve cell

Dendrites act to conduct the electrochemical signals received from other neural cells to the cell body and also play a vital role in integrating synaptic input and monitoring the extent of the action potential produced from the neurons. Dendrites always appear near the cell body. The axon is the smallest projection of a nerve cell that conducts electrical impulses, like dendrites. Axons are more of a receiver compared to dendrites and also make more contact with other cells, usually other neurons but sometimes muscles or gland cells.

The central nervous system (CNS), together with the peripheral nervous system (PNS), has a fundamental role in the control of behavior. The PNS consists of nerves and ganglia outside of the brain and spinal cord. Their function is mainly to connect the CNS to the limbs and organs. Radiating from the central nervous system is the peripheral nervous system, which has three parts to connect mainly to our senses and skin and muscles. To carry nerve impulses in different directions requires two groups of neurons. The sensory neurons are afferent neurons directed toward the CNS. The motor neurons are efferent neurons directed away from the CNS.

The Autonomic Nervous System

The autonomic nervous system works according to a plan. Sometimes you need one part of the system to function, but in other periods, it's important for a different part to kick in. As the name *autonomic nervous system* implies, the system works without any mental interaction, although occasionally, such as for breathing, the ANS works in tandem with the conscious mind. The ANS consists of three parts:

- the sympathetic branch
- the parasympathetic branch
- the enteric branch

The third branch, the enteric nervous system (ENS), manages every aspect of digestion, from the esophagus to the stomach, small intestine, and colon. But I will leave the ENS and concentrate on the more important two other nervous systems, the sympathetic nervous system and the parasympathetic nervous system.

The sympathetic nervous system:

- Is action-oriented
- Is always ready for fight
- Widens the lungs and increases blood flow

The parasympathetic nervous system:

- Slows down heart rate
- Redirects blood flow from legs to the gut
- Tranquillizes body activities

Since the sympathetic nervous system is action–oriented whereas the parasympathetic nervous system slows down the body, which do you prefer be operational when you go to bed for the night?

To simply demonstrate the difference between the two systems, imagine briskly walking in a park for half an hour. You have blood pumping from heart to lungs, and then out to your limbs. When you come home a little bit tired, you want some relief! You settle down on a sofa, and now your legs fly automatically up on a low table. What happens? Your blood is pumping back from your limbs. You are starting to feel more tired and soon you start yawning as you see the evening light. When you put up your legs, blood rushes away from them, which is a classic scenario for the parasympathetic nervous system reaction. Gravitational pull, like when you walk or run, is typically sympathetic activated. And that is why it is so important for us to shift from one nervous system to the other. We need some sort of switch to do just that. We will return to this scenario later.

Effects of Stimulation of the Autonomic Nervous System:

Organs	Sympathetic	Parasympathetic
Heart rate	Increased	Reduced
Heart strength	Increased	Reduced
Pupils	Dilated	Constricted
Lung, bronchial muscle	Relaxed	Contracted
Intestines, muscle activities	Reduced	Increased
Bladder, wall	Relaxed	Contracted
Bladder, sphincter	Contracted	Relaxed

Table 2. Effects of stimulation of the autonomic nervous system

The sympathetic nervous system activates the glands and organs that defend the body against attack and direct more blood to the muscles and the brain. This activates the thyroid and adrenal glands to provide energy for activities; to fight and to defend is the normal explanation. A normal mental reaction is to feel nervousness, stress, panic, or urgent counter reaction. The adrenalin rush is a product of the sympathetic system, which feels okay in the beginning, but will later cause fatigue and feeling exhausted. To be in a sympathetic state is not what you want when closing up for the day.

To change to parasympathetic activities is vital for people with a weak sleep capacity. The parasympathetic system is concerned with nourishing, healing, and regeneration of the body. It is an anabolic process to rebuild the body. The vital organs are the liver, pancreas, stomach, and intestines. To be in the parasympathetic nervous system as much as possible moves you into a healthy and healing state. To turn off and change from the "day" nervous system to the "night" system must be a key action to promote sleep.

Neurotransmitters

The whole chain of reactions in our very complex nervous system wouldn´t be possible without neurotransmitters; they are essential. Neurotransmitters are compounds that transmit signals from a neuron to target cells across a synapse. A synapse is a small gap or junction between two neurons or a neuron and a muscle. Release of neurotransmitters usually follows actions at the synapse. Neurotransmitters are synthesized from plentiful and simple compounds such as amino acids, which are easily available from the diet and which require only a small number of biosynthetic steps to convert. There are several types of neurotransmitters, and each one of them is responsible for some specific functions.

Important neurotransmitters:

Glutamate is used at the great majority of fast excitatory synapses in the brain and spinal cord. Glutamate is also used at most synapses that are increasing or decreasing in strength. Excessive glutamate release can lead to cell death.

GABA is used at the great majority of fast inhibitory synapses in virtually every part of the brain. Many sedative or tranquilizing drugs act by enhancing the effects of GABA.

Acetylcholine is distinguished as the transmitter at the neuromuscular junction connecting motor nerves to muscles. Acetylcholine also operates in many regions of the brain, but using different types of receptors. For us, this will be a key transmitter, due to its interacting capacity with motor nerve cells.

Dopamine has a number of important roles in the brain. Dopamine plays a critical role in the rewards system, and the dysfunction of the dopamine system is also implicated in Parkinson´s disease and schizophrenia.

Serotonin is a monoamine neurotransmitter. It is mostly produced by and found in the intestine (90 percent), and the remainder is in central nervous system neurons. It regulates appetite, sleep, memory and learning, and muscle contraction.

The Human Constitution

To have the wrong nervous system active in the evening without possessing a tool to switch to the other is not what you want when closing down for the night. If you are predisposed to an overactive nervous system, it will always be a struggle for you to calm down. Unfortunately, this is almost always the case if you have been fighting for better sleep for a long time—assuming, of course, that you can't find a natural reason. I believe that some people have more sleep problems by birth than others, and therefore have to find a solution of their own. Is it possible that most sleep-deprivation sufferers have had such a predisposition since birth? Is there an insomnia constitution to start with?

To answer that question you might go from the Western hemisphere and turn to the eastern direction. Since I'd worked part-time as an alternative therapist in the past and used these old medical laws frequently, I wanted to start with that clue. To search for solutions among old traditions of human constitutions or at least find out what these old archetypes of Eastern medical traditions shows us and to make the best solutions in the chase of better sleep.

Both Indian Ayurveda and Chinese acupuncture give us much information. Both "schools" are old and have certain fixed constitutions/archetypes for human mental and physical status. It has been shown several times that the old truth is coming back into use. Ayurveda and acupuncture have been adopted more and more by the medical establishment. More and more scientific proofs and reports point toward acceptance and give patients more selection when needed. The National Center for Complementary and Alternative Medicine (NCCAM) estimates that in the United States about 38 percent of adults use some form of complementary or alternative medicine. According to the 2007 National Health Interview Survey of 12,000 participants, alternative treatment is greater among women and those with higher levels of education and income.

Eastern philosophies have fixed human constitutions, which show in a very easy and simple way that there are at least two opposite forces against each other in the body. Of course, it makes no sense that in all these earth inhabitants, there are just two opposite poles to describe the human constitution. Imagine 7 billion people and put them all in or between those poles, and every soul will find its right place. By looking into Eastern philosophy, you get some answers, and it clearly shows that some people have more to fight about to achieve a perfect sleep. My meaning is just to give you a brief overlook so you will see with my eyes.

Old Indian Healing Truth

Ayurveda, the science of life, is a system of traditional medicine; it is practiced in many parts of the world as a form of alternative medicine. The earliest literature of Ayurveda appeared during the Vedic period, in the second millennium BCE continuing up to the sixth century BCE, based on literary evidence in India. The *Sushruta Samhita* and the *Charaka Samhita* were influential works on traditional medicine during this era. You can wonder what we had for medical knowledge in the Western world during the beginning of ayurvedic tradition.

My goal is not to dig deep into the latest research of ayurveda, but only to persuade readers to have an open mind and remind them that ayurveda is a very old school of medicine.

Ayurveda is grounded in a metaphysics that composes the universe of the human body. According to ayurveda, three regulatory principles, or *doshas*, are important for health because when they are balanced, the body is healthy.

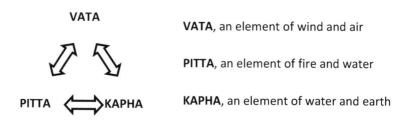

VATA, an element of wind and air

PITTA, an element of fire and water

KAPHA, an element of water and earth

Figure 6. The three doshas

The five great elements are within these doshas. Ayurveda holds that humans possess a unique combination of doshas. To describe them in an easy way, vata consists of everything light and fast, kapha is heavy and slow, and pitta is everything in between.

Vata

Vata is composed of wind and air, it governs all movements in the mind and body and must be kept in good balance. Too much vata leads to worry, insomnia, cramps, and constipation, theory says. Vata activates the nervous system, hearing, and speech; it can be expressed as enthusiasm and creativity. Vata wants to start things, to have several projects going on at the same time. Vata also controls the other two principles, pitta and kapha, and therefore it is the first dosha to be affected by disease. Old traditions claim that a weakness of vata in the constitution results in eighty diseases.

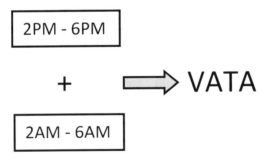

Figure 7. Vata dosha

Vata dominates in the first cycle from 2:00 p.m. to 6:00 p.m. and in the second cycle from 2:00 a.m. to 6:00 a.m. Unfortunately, when vata dominates to six o'clock in the morning, it means to get up before that time. Normally vata is very quick to awaken, and therefore it's preferable to follow the vata profile.

This seems to be a contradiction; vata starts at two o'clock, and shouldn't you be sleeping at that time? This question puzzled me for a period of time during the writing of this book. Then it struck me! At that time of night, you are normally very active if your REM sleep is intact. You are sleeping, but you are still very active. The blood that flows to the brain is twice as much during REM sleep compared to during the daytime. Can you believe it? So when the active vata dosha starts at two o'clock in the nighttime, it's exactly on schedule for REM sleep to start. Going to bed at ten o'clock, you have three to four hours to sleep through a deep sleep state, and then gradually change your sleep pattern to the lighter REM sleep. On the other hand, if you wake up from REM sleep, you normally do it in the middle of the night, which is in the beginning of vata period.

Pitta

Pitta is composed of fire and water, and thus governs all heat and metabolism. Pitta controls how we digest food, determine our sensory perceptions, and decide between right and wrong. Too much pitta can lead to anger, criticism, ulcers, rashes, and thinning of hair.

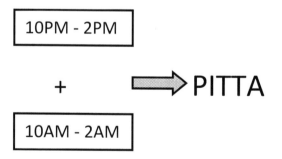

Figure 8. Pitta dosha

Pitta dominates in the first cycle from 10:00 p.m. until 2:00 p.m. and in the second cycle from 10:00 a.m. to 2:00 a.m. The first cycle shows that the most important meal is during lunchtime between ten and two o´clock.

Kapha

Kapha consists of earth and water. This element in the body provides for physical structure, such as maintaining body resistance, lubricating the joints, providing moisture to the skin, helping to heal wounds, supporting memory retention, and giving energy to the heart and lungs. Kapha is responsible for emotions of attachment, greed, and long-standing envy. Too much kapha leads to lethargy and weight gain, as well as congestion and allergies.

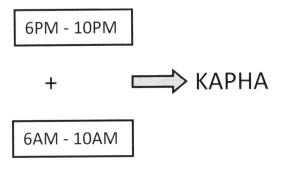

Figure 9. Kapha dosha

Kapha dominates in the first cycle from 6:00 p.m. to 10:00 p.m. and in the second cycle from 6:00 a.m. to 10:00 a.m. It is preferable that you follow the vata profile in the morning, but it's equally important to follow the kapha profile in the evening. Meaning; go to bed before ten o'clock, and you'll gain a great deal by having a boost of kapha sleeping and relaxation. A good sleeper has very significant influences from the kapha state.

Can it be coincidence that you should get to bed before ten o'clock to gain kapha's influence and get up before six o'clock to have a kick by vata? Anyway, it's something you should keep in mind. Even if you don't have a regular job at the moment, it's still essential to have some discipline. Remember, it is not only about how much you have been sleeping the night before; equally important is how many hours you had behind you, meaning when you got up in the morning to start the sleep clock.

Below I show you the differences between vata and kapha, because pitta is in the middle of their other and therefore not needed when to explain the opposite sleep forces of ayurveda.

The differences between vata and kapha are summarized below:

Vata	Earth inhabitant	Kapha
• Activated CNS		• Body structure
• Active		• Grounded
• Restless		• Relaxed
• Fast		• Slow
• Insomnia		• Good sleeper
• Cold		• Warm
• Dry		• Oily

Figure 10 Vata and Kapha summarized

To place all earth inhabitants in between those poles are of course a gigantic generalization, but some people are nearer vata and therefore inherent certain difficulties. In ayurveda theory, every human body consists of vata, pitta, and kapha; the problem is to have all three in balance. Sickness comes when one of the doshas is in excess. Ayurveda is very clear that insomnia comes from a vata imbalance. Vata has both wind and air, which is very light and has a low resistance to disturbance. If your body is turned in the vata direction, you have a very active mind and body. The problem is to shut vata down or reduce its activity.

Ayurveda also focuses on exercise, yoga, meditation, and massage. For diagnosis, the patient is to be questioned, and all five senses are to be employed. Two researchers have given ayurveda great recognition in the United States and the Western world through Western medical documentation. Frank John Ninivaggi, MD, of Yale

University School of Medicine, researched and outlined its various postulates in one major textbook suitable to Western academic science: Ayurveda: A Comprehensive Guide to Traditional Indian Medicine for the West. The National Institute of Ayurvedic Medicine, established by Dr. Scott Gerson (located in Brewster, NY) is also an example of an ayurveda research institute.

Acupuncture, a Chinese healing Therapy

Acupuncture is a treatment method that originated more than three thousand years ago in China, during the Xia Dynasty (2000 to 1500 BC), and it is still practiced in many parts of the world today. The method is commonly practiced as a routine treatment in China, Japan, Korea, and Taiwan. Since the late 1970s, it has also gained popularity in the Western world.

Acupuncture, a traditional Chinese needle therapy, has become widely used for the relief of headache or pain in any form. There is evidence from meta-analyses of randomized controlled trials (RCTs), explained by Rapson and Banner, to support the fact that acupuncture relieves chronic low back and neck pain. They conclude: Acupuncture has a sound physiological basis and is safe and effective for the management of musculoskeletal, inflammatory, and neuropathic pain. Knowledge of acupuncture can make self-treatment with TENS devices a useful tool for pain management, including cancer pain

Acupuncture is among the best known of complementary and alternative therapies for use in humans, but it is also in widespread use in animals. Still, it has been only in recent years, a couple of decades ago, since the medical establishment in Sweden said yes to treating pain with acupuncture. About one million American patients receive alternative medicine treatment, and there are approximately seventeen thousand acupuncturists in the United States.

Insomnia and *Stretch to Sleep*™-Program

The Theory of Acupuncture

The practice of acupuncture consists of inserting fine, solid needles into selected body locations, which are called acupuncture points. Classic texts describe 365 points located systematically on meridians, or channels of energy. According to the concepts of Chinese medicine, disease and pain are the result of imbalance of yin and yang, and acupuncture treatment aims to restore that balance.

Yin refers to the feminine aspect of life—nourishing, receptive, and soft.

Yang is the male counterpart—hard, dominant, and energetic.

If you compare the two element theories—ayurveda and acupuncture—you find ayurveda is much easier to understand, and its five elements are more natural to comprehend. Acupuncture, on the other hand, has the advantage that all of the points are very specific and easy to use.

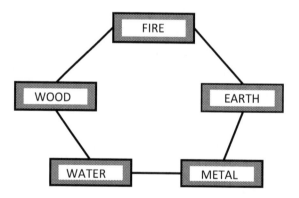

Figure 11. The five elements

Imbalances in the flow of qi among the meridians, organs, and the five elements are the cause of disease, pain, and susceptibility to illness. The movement among these opposing forces, named qi, is considered to be the essential element in the healing system of Traditional Chine Medicine, TCM. Inserting needles at key points along these meridians balances such factors as heat, cold, dampness, and dryness. The acupoints are located at sites that have a high density of neurovascular structures and are generally between or at the edges of muscle groups.

The ancient Chinese believed that qi is the vital energy or life force, and all that matters in the universe appears by the movements and mutations of qi. There are fourteen major meridians, including twelve regular double (each side of the body) and two main center meridians in the body. The concept of yin and yang is the generalization of the two opposite aspects in related objects and phenomena in the natural world. Some yin-yang examples include tranquility and motion, lower and upper body, and the parasympathetic and sympathetic system.

The differences between yin and yang can be summarized as follows:

Yang:	Earth inhabitants	Yin:
• Active		• Resting
• Light		• Dark
• Fast		• Slow
• Hot		• Cold

Figure 12. Yang and Yin summarized

For optimal function, your body needs to have good balance between the yin and the yang, but this is not always the scenario. To take advantage of acupuncture theory is to use some of the points to slow down the yang and to speed up the yin. To feel yang at its peak in the evening, instead of lacy yin, can destroy the whole night. The main purpose of this information is for you to understand what is in charge and why the body cannot rest.

An example of a sudden imbalance is the following: you have been sleeping a reasonable time, but suddenly wake up hot and bathed in sweat. That is typical yang proving its capability, and yang can be very strong and persistent. When you're suddenly awake and hot, your thoughts are impossible to stop. Your mind functions at its best when you're warm.

Summary of the Human Constitutions

As you can see in the table that follows, the left column and the right column have almost the same information from top to bottom. This is just a brief clarification and generalization as to what you can find in the different types of human classifications or constitutions. There are surely a bunch of contrary opinions about this information, but I want to show you that there are similarities among us. This chapter about human constitutions shows a key point to the problem that good sleepers do not have. The thing is, good sleepers don't have to do anything. They don't have think of such things as "sleep hygiene." They don't know what it means. Their ability to sleep is determined by a very high activity of the sleep hormone melatonin, which takes care of everything. They can sleep standing, or at least even when watching a good movie.

The left column is a strong contrast to the right column. The key problem when trying to sleep is to slow down activity and to shift the nervous system. Almost all insomnia treatments aim to reduce tension and to slow down yang activity or shift to the kapha state. The complaints from people with severe sleep difficulties say that they can't come to rest. They can't shut down their bodies. How do you find the switch? Is there a way to switch the nervous system to find relief? The table below shows the archetypes, a very strong generalization of human constitutions. To show you a brief explanation of Eastern philosophy I want you to notes that according to these old traditions there are already pointed out weaknesses for certain ailments or symptoms. It seems that some inhabitants already been born with weak sleep abilities. This is a brief explanation, but it is meant to help to understand what needs to be done. We are all different; therefore we need to find a small truth of our own to find a cure to a tricky situation.

When some people, good sleepers, pointed out that it is just to relax and sleep, you know now, it isn't that easy. Some people are born to struggle with their sleep abilities. To find an ailment to improve your sleep is to make a counterattack toward bad influences to your body system, which has probably haunted you for a long time or forever.

Insomnia-constitution	Sleep-constitution
• Difficult to rest • Stressed • Sympathetic reactive	• Relaxed • Sleep everywhere • Parasympathetic reactive
Vata-constitution	**Kapha-constitution**
• Nervous system • Restless • Fast • Insomnia • Sympathetic reactive	• Body structure • Relaxed • Slow • Good sleeper • Parasympathetic reactive
Yang-constitution	**Yin-constitution**
• Active • Light • Fast • Hot • Sympathetic reactive	• Resting • Dark • Slow • Cold • Parasympathetic reactive

Table 3 Summary of the human constitutions

Exercise and Stretching

To achieve most from S2S-Program I want to pick up an important issue, before I present the program in detail. Exercise has been part of my whole life, and it is more or less a habit of mine. And I do think if you hold your body in trim you gain more in stretching ability, a trained body is more prone to gain more from stretching, then untrained. Therefore it should be a habit of yours just to keep on exercise, whatever you do. And for many reasons, exercise might be something good for your sleep, not just for overall benefits, such as condition for your lung and heart etc. If you continue training for a long time, it's hard to stop, because you know that the effort to start from the beginning is harder than just carrying on.

For many people, stretching is essential, and they practice it almost every day. For instance, looking at athletics, stretching is an important part of daily training. It is used in the beginning and the ending of sessions to maintain accurate muscle status, and reduce tenseness of muscles, whatever the athlete is practicing. Of course, you don't have to be a top athlete to use stretching. But how many people practice stretching regularly and how many use stretching before going to bed? I mean, after a whole day of work, you don't need to stretch? At least I think, there are considerable amount of people out there needing a good stretch. I admit that for some people—those with mostly soft muscle and over flexed joints—stretching isn't for them. I suppose that the answer for those people is more training without stretching.

Stretching can be used for a variety of purposes and as a method to reduce muscle soreness following activity. For instance, neck pain is a significant contributor to worldwide disability and poses a considerable financial burden according to doctors. Up to 70 percent of the population will experience an episode of neck pain at some point in their lives, and 15 percent of the population will experience chronic neck pain (Childs et. al). Approaches suggest that the inclusion of stretching and strengthening exercises for acute and chronic mechanical neck disorders results in a favorable response. Change in lifestyle and inclusion of physical activity decreased neck pain. Other lifestyle modifications that complement a general increase in physical activity have been demonstrated to be effective. Common physical characteristics are shared by patients with neck and low back pain. Although stretching exercises alone have demonstrated an ability to decrease neck pain, other studies suggest a combination of strength training and stretching exercises for chronic neck pain. In a randomized controlled trial (Ylinen et. al) assessed the effectiveness of manual therapy procedure implemented twice a week compare with a stretching regimen performed 5 times a week in those with non-specific neck pain. The authors concluded that the low-cost of stretching exercise should include in the initial treatment, although, there were a significant small differences in favor for manual therapy.

There are many benefits to be gained from regular stretching. Normally mentioned are the following:

- Increased flexibility
- Decreased injuries
- Improved posture
- Sport improvements
- Stress relief

Increased flexibility is obviously a benefit of regular stretching and usually the reason that people start a stretching program. Being flexible can help to prevent injuries. Stretching has been used in the warm-up process for many years. It is thought that having flexible muscles can prevent acute injuries by gently stretching the muscle through its range before exercise. Many sports obviously require high levels of flexibility, for example, athletics and gymnastics. In order for muscles to be healthy, they must be flexible. Muscle tightness is often associated with stress—we tend to tighten up when stressed. Stretching relaxes these muscles and you at the same time!

Results of a randomized trial (Bello-Hass) suggest that moderate resistance training and stretching exercises helped patients with amyotrophic lateral sclerosis (ALS) maintain function and improved quality of life versus a group offered usual care. The role of exercise in patients with ALS has been controversial, but recent evidence has suggested low- or moderate-intensity exercise may have some benefit in maintaining function. In the study by Malliaropoulos and associates, the group that performed a more intensive stretching program was found to regain full active knee extension compared with the uninjured side earlier than the group that performed a less intensive stretching program. Time needed for rehabilitation was also significantly shorter in the intensive stretching group than in the less intensive stretching group.

Different training can serve different purposes. The older you get, the more you gain from maintaining a variety of exercises; and it is a huge advantage compared to beginners if you have kept exercising from an early age,. Appropriate physical activity also enhances relaxation. There is evidence that regular physical activity can reduce stress and anxiety. Numerous people report an improvement in their mood following appropriate physical activity. That is what people refer to as the mind-body relationship.

When you at last retire after a whole life of struggle, it can be sudden and very direct. For some, it's okay; they have been waiting for that special moment for a long time. Others, though, want to keep on working. I suppose sometimes it has to do with what comes after retirement—grandchildren, hobbies, and so on. Everybody needs a break, a period without work and a regular schedule, but after a while, it can be difficult for you to sleep. What is there to get you tired? For instance, a muscle needs exercise to be strong; otherwise, it goes rigid. It's like a motor that is not looked after. All systems shut down. Physical inactivity and sedentary living contribute to a decrease in independence and the onset of many chronic diseases. This leads to significantly increasing health and social care costs. Physically active lifestyles can help delay the onset of physical frailty and disease, thereby significantly reducing these health and social care costs.

According to science, long-term benefits in almost all aspects of psychological functioning have been observed following periods of extended physical activity. They include:

- Improved mental health
- Contribution in the treatment of several mental illnesses
- Decreased depression
- Lessening of anxiety neurosis

As far as cognitive improvements are concerned, regular physical activity may help postpone age-related declines in the central nervous system processing speed and reaction time. When retired, a large proportion of older adults gradually adopt a sedentary lifestyle, which eventually threatens to reduce independence and self-sufficiency. Activity is important not only for sleep quality, but also for social activity. Participation in appropriate physical activity can help empower older individuals and assist them in playing a more active role in society.

It has been estimated that there are 4.5 million gym members in the United Kingdom, but only 27 percent of them exercise on a regular basis. That is to put money in the bin. From a population of 62 million plus people, only 1.6 percent has the habit to visit a gym on a regular basis. So, in the United Kingdom, there are millions of gym members, but there are surely more other millions of people who are not visiting gym facilities at all. There is so much to gain with regular exercise, from a wide range of perspectives. Overall physical activity levels decrease with aging, and only an estimated 50 percent of all persons who initiate an exercise program continue the habit for more than six months. Normally it takes a trigger, like a life-threatening condition, to cause people to make exercise an important part of their lives.

Exercise commonly refers to a specific plan of fitness activities that are designed for a specified purpose. Such a plan is often developed by an instructor, but it can be a self-made plan. To help your body system most, activity should be performed for at least thirty to sixty minutes, four to six times weekly, or thirty minutes on most days of the week, according to Amer Suleman, MD, Medical City Dallas Hospital. Exercise goals should include both the heart system and your muscle and tendon system. A heart workout program means aerobic activities, such as bicycling, walking, swimming, and so forth. Resistive exercises using free weights or standard equipment restore your muscular tone. Resistive training should be performed two or three times per week. For adults, it is most important to develop good muscle tone and strengthen the body.

Maximal muscle contraction force and muscle mass are both reduced during the natural aging process, and long-term training may be used to attenuate this age-related loss in muscle function and muscle size. For some elderly individuals, the loss in muscle function may represent a serious risk for loss of freedom or independence. The big picture is a lifestyle of physical activity from childhood throughout the adult years to increase health and longevity, which have been proclaimed by science authorities for ages to benefit from exercise. Even a brisk walk as a physical activity or exercise habit promotes health benefits. Resistance training is recommended by a number of health promotion organizations for its effects to strengthen muscle mass, among other parameters. For elderly individuals, resistance training is even more important, for maintenance of flexibility and the quality of life.

Exercise offers the following benefits:

- Improved insulin sensitivity
- Decreased blood pressure and low-density lipoprotein
- Increased high-density lipoprotein levels

Saving your muscle size late in life may prevent the normal age-related loss in skeletal muscle mass and protect against the development of metabolic conditions such as reduced glucose tolerance and impaired insulin sensitivity (type II diabetes). It seems extremely important to keep a lifelong training habit that can reduce the age-related decline in muscle fiber.

You have heard for years that it is important to practice endurance training, to work your heart, but that is not the whole truth. A study on elderly individuals suggests that resistance training is superior to endurance training in delaying the age-related loss in muscle mass. It is especially effective in counteracting the preferential reduction in type II fiber area that is typically observed with aging. Muscle mass, as well as maximal contractile muscle strength and power, are reduced with aging. For elderly individuals, the loss in muscle mechanical function may represent a serious risk for loss of independence. Long-term training may be used to attenuate this age-related loss in muscle function and muscle size. Mechanical muscle performance seems to be retained at a higher level in aged individuals exposed to lifelong strength training. I also believe for sure that a strengthened muscle promotes overall sleeping quality. But there may be times where this issue needs extra care and thinking. For instance, a stiff muscle does not promote sleep.

More and more evidence claims that moderate-intensity activities are not enough, because vigorous-intensity activities may have greater benefit for reducing cardiovascular disease and premature mortality than moderate-intensity physical activity. So you can only reduce time in a training center if you are prepared to incorporate intensity in the program. To just sit on a bike, perhaps watching a TV, is not good enough; you have to perform. "Resistance exercise training increases muscular strength and is currently prescribed by major health organizations for improving health and fitness," wrote Jonatan R. Ruiz and colleagues from Karolinska Institutes in Huddinge, Sweden

A study by McManama Ackermann and associates showed that exercise may improve RLS (Restless Legs Syndrome) symptoms. Twenty-three participants completed the trial. The exercise group was prescribed a conditioning program of aerobic and lower-body resistance training three days per week. The prescribed exercise program was effective in improving the symptoms of RLS at the end of the twelve weeks. Future studies are needed to further address the effects of exercise on the symptoms of RLS. The current study results are promising, but larger studies are necessary before exercise is routinely prescribed for RLS, the researchers concluded.

Exercise can have, from my experience, direct good or bad impact on the quality of sleep. But in the long run, it has positive influences on the whole body system, at the end interacting throughout every nerve synapse to maintain balanced homeostasis. Regular exercise makes muscles work and improves blood supply. Cold muscles or inactive ones make it harder to stretch. If you work too hard at the wrong time, it has the opposite effects. As I mentioned before, early in life, for a good sleeper, exercise doesn't matter; but later in life, the situation could change.

Stretching and RLS

I want to give you a brief explanation of this topic due to my feeling that many sufferers don't think they have any problem with it; many people suffer light complaints (like myself), of which they aren't fully aware. With my S2S-program, you can find some relief in both the restless legs syndrome and sleep problems at the same time.

The first clinical description of RLS is generally attributed to the seventeenth-century British anatomist and physician Thomas Willis, who described the syndrome and was also the first to suggest a treatment. In more modern times, the term *restless legs syndrome* was used initially in the mid-1940s by Swedish neurologist Karl A. Ekbom in a presentation of fifty-three cases.

Prevalence and Epidemiology (Allen):

- Affects approximately 3% - 10 % of the general population (US)
- Occurrence: female 1.5 to 2 times more than male
- More common with increasing age

Do you have uncomfortable sensations within your legs and therefore a feeling to move your legs in response to these sensations? Well, then you belong to a large group of people with similar symptoms. These sensations feel like restlessness in your limbs, and they were conveniently named restless legs syndrome (RLS). RLS has been found to produce a chronic sleep loss more severe than almost any other condition, and it impairs quality of life as much or more than other chronic diseases. Several factors have contributed to the recent attention given to RLS. It is recognized now as a neuralgic movement disorder, often associated with a sleep complaint. RLS can cause dramatic distress, greatly disturbed quality of life, and profoundly disrupted sleep.

IRLSSG, International Restless Legs Syndrome Study Group, stated for primary RLS as follow:

- An urge to move, usually due to uncomfortable sensations that occur primarily in the legs
- Motor restlessness, expressed as activity, that relieves the urge to move
- Worsening of symptoms by relaxation
- Variability over the course of the day-night cycle, with symptoms worse in the evening and early in the night

Patients with RLS have a characteristic difficulty in trying to describe their symptoms, doctors say; they may report sensations such as an almost irresistible urge to move the legs, which is not painful but can lead to significant physical and emotional

110

disability. RLS patients typically described it as being on pins and needles, a creeping feeling, or a crawling sensation. Often, patients simply state or describe the sensations as uncomfortable and being deep within the leg, rather than on the surface. Some patients have learned that a counter stimulus, such as rubbing their legs, may provide relief. Most alerting stimulation will reduce the symptoms, including very hot or cold baths.

Circadian rhythm variation not only interferes with sleep, but also intervenes with your system and gives unpleasant symptoms. Often, symptoms are relieved after 5:00 a.m., like many sleep complaints, fading away in the beginning of the morning due to the circadian rhythm. However, in more severe cases, symptoms can be present throughout the day without circadian variation. In most cases, this sleep disorder is treated with drugs. People who suffer from this sleep disorder usually have to stay on their medications for the rest of their lives.

Stretch Release

At home after work, you take care of your home duties. There's still quite some time left of the evening. You feel tense. You try to relax, sitting in front of the TV and looking at your favorite show or reading a chapter from a new book. You feel tired and tense. You're looking at your watch; soon it's time to go to bed. "Will my sleep work tonight?" you wonder. You enter your bed in a sleepy, but not relaxed, mood. The same story tonight comes into your mind. "Where is my switch for sleep?" You think desperately after an hour of clear wakefulness. Tense muscles can put us over the edge. What to do? If you have tense muscles, meaning short muscles, just stretch them out. You say, "I do that every time I work out, two times a week." Sorry, that's not enough. Even if you work out every day and have a proper stretch, it doesn't ensure that you will be relaxed in the evening.

Stretching is for the moment. Is it important to do stretching exercises even if you didn't do a workout after your daily job? Yes, of course! Even if you just sit in one spot eight hours a day, you get stiff. Remember, muscles get stiff in time. If you have been sitting and working with your computer the whole day, you have to do something about that.

What can we gain from a relaxed muscle? The first benefit is that you feel relaxed. Why? Because your muscles are more soft and not tense. Well, it depends when you are doing your exercise, what time during the day or evening. Hopefully you go from work to your gym, do your workout or spinning, and then end with a stretch. After a hard workout, it feels good to do a finishing stretch. You feel relaxed, at the moment.

Even if you have a physically varied job, you need relaxation. Perhaps you can't complain at all; everything is great, except you feel a little bit stressed. You enjoy every moment—positive stress—but when you come home, you find it hard to relax. You sit down after your home duties and watch TV but still feel not relaxed. Some people have by birth, a relaxed body, but you aren't among them. Have faith! You are not alone. There are bunches of sisters and brothers who share the same destiny.

Imagine that you have an energy flow around you, in you, constantly. This flow is working perfectly when your body is in balance. What happens if that energy is stopped or choked? Well, your nice flow wouldn't support you, and it's the same when going to sleep at night. If your flow is out of order, what happens with your ability to rest? You cannot! What happens in the figure on the left if your strong leg muscle is tense? Do you have a nice flow? No, I don't think so. To a person with weak sleep, everything counts. Bring your body into balance! Do your stretch for a while and change your energy patterns.

Believe me, a tense body is best relaxed by physical intervention. Mental relaxation is a great thing, but not to start with.

Postulate

Body tension is released by physical stretching of muscles.

I don't mean this as the only solution for bad sleep, but surely it is a good start. You might say that sleeping pills have "helped" before. Isn't it strange that so many are seeking help from that type of medication, and still have not been cured? They have been a help for the moment, but a cure? No! I know sometimes it is necessary to use antidepressants or benzodiazepines. But there are other alternatives to consider. Is there something equal that you share with your sisters and brothers? I think there is. Your constitutions are similar to each other's. You are more prone to take in external stimuli, which is disadvantageous for you.

Nature is created by two forces fighting each other or working together—bad or good, strong or weak, long or short, warm or cold, dark or light, givers or takers. Is it impossible that it could be the same in the human constitution?

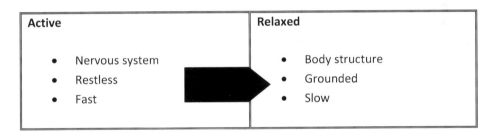

Active	Relaxed
• Nervous system	• Body structure
• Restless	• Grounded
• Fast	• Slow

S2S-Program Blueprint Symptoms

Now we come to a state of truth. What can I offer for sufferers of bad sleep? The Stretch to Sleep Program, S2S Program, is meant to be a healing program for people with sleeping difficulties. You can't expect to find a single aid to promote good sleep. People fly to the moon and back, but humanity still has problems finding enough peace to sleep. Yes, it is easy to grab some pills, but to do it in harmony with your body is another story. There is a huge amount of books already written about sleep and sleep-related problems, but I hope to bring some new ideas and findings to support this group of sufferers.

To gain the most from the S2S program, you should fit into the profile below.

S2S-Program Blueprint Symptoms:

- Feel restless during day or evening
- Have stiff legs and muscles
- Never feel restored
- Always in a hurry

Those five symptoms are not very hard to find in our society today. Such people abound among us; and even if there are a lot of people who sleep very well despite the five problems above, you know by the statistics presented earlier that there are many sufferers out there. You already know what type I'm talking about. I am searching for a certain constitution, a human blueprint type, to fit my S2S-program profile. I am the first to admit this is a huge generalization, but the S2S program is meant to fit a specific type of group.

S2S-Program Blueprint Constitution:

- Vata dominant
- Yang dominant

The fundamental problem for most people is a lack of ability to rest. They feel that their body is too excited, stiff, and not ready to sleep. Here is the main task to solve. Therefore, my first mission is to take care of this problem straightaway. In the market today there are many companies that want to help you to calm down with relaxation programs, focused only through mental aids. Of course, this is not totally wasted money, but it not efficient enough. It is in the wrong order. You have to begin at square one. Your mental state must come after the main relaxation from the physical intervention of your body. So what is there in your body that cannot be released by mental force? Yes, quite right—your muscles! We have more or less six hundred muscles throughout our bodies, and for some reason, they can't be relaxed on command. I know what you're thinking: "I can relax whenever I want." But that is not true. If you have a problem in sleeping, you cannot relax enough, or at least that is the starting point to begin with. There are no other methods that can give you faster releasing ability.

Postulate:

You can't relax a body mentally if your physical body is stiff.

To be fit and for your muscles to function properly, you need to work out on a regular basic. You need to do something to shape up your system. There is evidence that regular physical activity can reduce stress and anxiety. Numerous people report improvement in their mood state following appropriate physical activity. Science says that appropriate physical activity enhances relaxation. That is what is meant by the mind-body relationship.

Even so, more and more evidence claims that moderate activities are not enough, that vigorous-intensity activities may have greater benefit for reducing cardiovascular disease and premature mortality than moderate physical activity. Even for those with an insomnia constitution, exercise will be beneficial for their overall health condition, but for their sleep status, too much vigorous activity can be devastating. If you work out on a regular basis, pay attention to how stiff your muscles really are. Muscles are key issues in the theory of S2S, so we'll keep on this subject for a while. Is there any difference between types of muscle fibers?

Skeletal Muscle

Everybody has had some extended experience of muscles, even if they've never been on a track field. You just live your life needing muscle strength, and sooner or later, you've got a sore spot, pain in different parts of the body, for some reason. Even if you don't use your body, for instance, at work, you have reminders from your muscles. Using your muscles can give you pain, and not using them can equally give pain or soreness. Briefly, you need muscles just to be alive. And there are a few characteristics of muscles to keep in mind:

- Excitability; respond to stimuli (e.g., nervous impulses)
- Contractility; able to shorten in length
- Extensibility; stretch when pulled
- Elasticity; tend to return to original shape and length after contraction or extension

These four characteristics are highly important and interesting when you are starting the S2S program, and you can receive self-experience right away. I want to spotlight two of them: (1.) Muscles respond to stimuli, and (2.) Muscles stretch when pulled. These are what we gain a lot of points from when starting the S2S program. I'm sure many people have been active in some way and therefore are using their muscles. Even if you just have a nice walk or go out with your dog, you are doing something and using a bunch of muscles. You must admit, it is a nice feeling. By using muscles, you maintain the following functions:

- Motion
- Maintenance of posture
- Heat production

Muscle = Stress Pole Basin

Whether you are working, exercising, or just being alive, your muscles need taking care of, like you do with a car. Car owners know that they have to spend time and money for optimum longevity of the car. Muscles need exercise; otherwise they shrink. On the other hand, a worked muscle, or even worse, a worn-out muscle, tends to get stiff with time. For instance, for some people, their muscles have overactive potential. For a group of people, their muscles are like a stress pole basin and give wrong signals to the CNS. When a big muscle, for instance, in a leg is stressed, your brain thinks it is time for action and no time for a nap. But, of course, for a good sleeper, this makes no sense at all. Don't misunderstand me; stiff people do sleep, but this book is not for them.

Postulate

Tense or hard muscle = Sympaticus reactive

Muscles features

There are two important biologic features to keep track of muscles.

- Muscle spindle
- Golgi tendon organ

Muscle Spindle

Muscle spindles are sensory receptors within the belly of a muscle and are aligned parallel to extrafusal muscle fibers, composed of three to twelve intrafusal muscle fibers, and primarily detect changes in the length of this muscle. They convey length information to the central nervous system via sensory neurons. This information can be processed by the brain to determine the position of body parts. The responses of muscle spindles to changes in length also play an important role in regulating the contraction of muscles.

Golgi Tendon Organ

The Golgi tendon organ is a proprioceptive sensory receptor organ that is located at the insertion of skeletal muscle fibers into the tendons of skeletal muscle. It provides the sensory component of the Golgi tendon reflex. In a Golgi tendon reflex, skeletal muscle contraction causes the muscle to simultaneously lengthen and relax. This reflex is an inverse of the stretch reflex. Though muscle tension is increasing during the contraction, alpha motor neurons in the spinal cord supplying the muscle are inhibited. However, antagonistic muscles are activated.

Both these muscle organs are important features for measuring activity of muscles and for the brain to have a close checkup. That means if there is a tension and stiffness in big leg muscles, those organs find out and send a signal to the CNS. What's the fuss? Well, it's crucial. If you have tension and want to go to sleep, you probably can't, because the CNS didn't get the right signal to shift the nervous system. Your stress release organ is the Golgi tendon organ.

To be at your prime, all systems in your body (lymphatic, cardiovascular, nervous, etc.) should be in balance. For some people, they are. Very old and healthy persons are blessed with high performance-activated bodies, with all functions working properly. It's not likely to find a very old man or woman saying, "I've slept poorly all my life, despite my age." No, if a person is blessed with a high quality of sleep, there is much to gain in life, for life. Can you see any similarity to your life situations at the moment? You normally are highly active, with stiff and hard muscles and always on the run. You want something happening all the time, but can't pull the brake when it is needed. Is it hard to understand that when bedtime comes in the evening, you are highly active? You don't have the key to change, to shut down your engine (body).

Postulate

> Stretch muscles >
>
> Golgi tendon organ goes into action and sends a report to the CNS.

In your insomnia constitution, it will be harder to sleep; you have to make some effort to shift or change. As you know now, you're not put in this world to be the best sleeper. Two opposite forces are fighting to win: day versus night, or in medical terms, nervous Sympaticus versus nervous Parasympaticus. We are born with different abilities, and every person is individualistic.

For a person with an insomnia sleep pattern, sleep doesn't come naturally. You have to make it appear naturally—not unnaturally, like with sleeping pills. You want to wake up and still have a clear mind. To have a healthy sleep without drowsiness the next day must be the ultimate goal. Fortunately, these days, medically trained persons are more prone to take help from alternative treatments. Doctors are reducing their prescriptions of sleeping drugs, to the benefit of their patients.

Your body is what you can work with; your body is your laboratory! Even so, you can feel hopeless sometimes, but don't give up; there must be an answer for every question. There are numerous muscles to take under consideration. Which one is most important? Where do I start? To begin, you gain almost every time you stretch, if you are healthy in the area you are working with. First of all: the bigger the muscle you work with, the more you gain from stretching.

To practice stretching means you receive more benefits than only improved sleep quality. To relax a muscle means more blood supply to the area. Your tendons work more accurately. You get a huge release of the area around your stomach. When you work regularly with the S2S program, you will notice several signs you have not been aware of before.

Postulate

> The S2S program gives you more benefits than just sleep improvement.

Do you need to do the S2S program every evening? Is it enough just to stretch after your workout, and not before sleep? No, it isn't. Your muscle status is for the moment. If we talk about a chronic condition, such as a sickness, then you can have it for a lifetime. A healthy muscle, though, needs attention; think of your muscles as your best friends. A muscle loses its tone in a matter of hours. But muscles have good memories. If you haven't done a workout for a period of time, you can easily come up to the same level in no time. A muscle not only loses strength; it goes stiff rapidly. Every person is different, but having stiff muscles is highly characteristic for your insomnia constitution.

My opinion is that you can gain a lot of benefits from exercise on a regular basis. In fact, science says that those persons who have been active since early in life show better overall health. Exercise will boost and pump up your system, as well as get the blood moving in your body and muscles. A good spin-off effect of a regular training program is that warm, trained muscles are much easier to stretch than non-exercised muscles.

Postulate

> A worked muscle is easier to stretch than a non-exercised muscle.

However, working out several times a week without stretching will not improve your sleeping skills; it might go the other direction. Even if you are doing stretching exercises regularly after training, it's not enough. Training lifts your overall health level, but it does not improve your sleep—not for everyone. I can't point out more clearly that stretching is vital for your sleep.

It's a biological fact that your muscles tend to get stiffer every minute in the 24/7 cycle, even without any work. The older you get, the more rigid muscles give you functional problems in life, and for sure, sleeping abilities are reduced.

Postulate

> A stretched muscle goes stiff with time and age;
>
> stretching ability is for the moment

The time has come to start with the S2S program. This method is easy to learn for almost everybody, but for some, one or two exercises can be too much. Some exercises are essential for the whole program to succeed. So those persons not proceeding with the total S2S program might find it a disappointment.

The tone of the lower extremities determines the degree of switching. You can easily pick up signs from your bowels, like a gurgling sound or a small vibrating feeling. That is a good sign, because it shows that something is released in that area. Blocked energy now is free, and you can make better function of that body part.

Blocked energy $\Rightarrow$ Stretching $\Rightarrow$ Free energy

This first released muscle can give you a good picture of what you gain. You should have had the first yeaning, and in this state, you might feel the first relaxation spreading in your body. Para Sympaticus is now starting to push, which making you feel tired is coming through. The switch of the nervous system has started.

Stretching ⟹ Switch to Para Sympaticus NS

Again, this is not supposed to be a yoga lesson. But there are, of course, similarities throughout the S2S program. The S2S program has been adapted to a modern life for people on the run who want to achieve fast and safe relaxation before going to bed and therefore a better sleep quality and healthier life.

Those exercises promote not only a good sleep, but it also helps you loosen up blocked parts of your bowels; thanks to exercise, those blocked parts will be dissolved. Leg movements have a lot to do with how well your intestine works. If you're not walking around every now and then, your intestine work slows down. That's why elderly people have problems with constipation, among other health problems. But you can have the contrary scenario, and work and run too much in life, mostly at work. That is what we call in modern terms stress. What happens is that your body is charged with negative energy, which is stored in your muscles. This negative energy is blocking your body, and your stress hormone is pumping through your body at a high level. When you have reached a high stress level, all your muscles and tendons are very hard and stiff, and your body is not working properly. So the primary goal is to loosen up your stress and shift the nervous system.

To work with the S2S program, you need some time before bedtime. Make this a good habit every evening before going to bed. It will only take twenty minutes, but those will be the best-invested minutes in your life. A lot of people take everything for granted. They think: Why should I stretch for twenty minutes when I can take a sleeping pill in just a fraction of that time? My only answer is, it is better to be addicted to a good habit than to some destructive one. You can start the S2S-1 exercise before you enter your bedroom. I used to begin my program when looking at the TV. Be sure you're not watching a very exciting movie or something, because it could be hard to turn it off. Sometimes my legs have gone sleepy or numb, but that is not anything disturbing; just take it easy for a while. Remember, stretching is valuable only for the moment.

Now, I have given you the theoretical keys to understand the S2S program. Why? When? Soon we can get started on the practical exercises. And as I told you, big muscles are preferable. You have more to gain from working big muscles! To get your overall energy to spark—blood vessels, nerve endings, and so on—we should concentrate on the lower body, your legs. But, of course, when we finish the lower part, I find no reason not to continue to the upper part. There are some key areas where you can gain benefits. I mean, how many people haven't had any problems with the neck, arms, or shoulders? For sleep status, the lower part of the body is essential. If you don't want to do the whole program, at least do the first part.

The biggest muscle is situated in the lower part of your body to support standing or running. You find all vital organs in the torso, but nevertheless, they support each other. For us, it is essential to start to release yin and to bring down, to conquer yang. So that is our first strategy move: start with your legs in the chase of sleep.

Postulate

> Release the tension of your legs to promote yin activity.

And at last:

If you never stretched in your life or work out at in fitness center take it easy to start with. Stretching is not for all. If your joints/muscles already are soft this is not for you. If you got a weakness/injury, don't do stretching, but at least start the program and feel for yourself.

Now is time for action. Next chapter I show you what I feel is right stretch moves to achieve most when going to bed. Take your time and good luck.

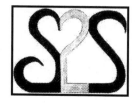

Part 4

S2S Program

in Practice

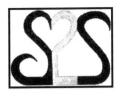

S2S-1: Thighs

M. Quadriceps Femoris or M. Rectus Femoris

As the name hints, this muscle consists of a group of four muscles. The thighs have the biggest muscles in the body, to support movement and transportation. The front of the thigh, M. Quadriceps femoris, gains the most from a stretching exercise. It's a big, strong bunch of four muscles; take it easy if it's your first time.

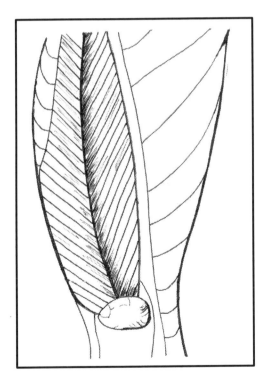

Function: Stretches the knee joint, bending the hip joint.

Tense muscle gives: pain or ache in the lower back or pain over and around the knee joints.

Important! Don't do this exercise if you have an unstable knee joint or a knee that has been operated on.

Figure 13. M Quadriceps femoris

125

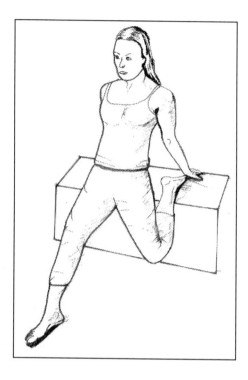

Figure 14. Thigh stretch

Implementation

Stretch your thigh when hold your foot in a firm positions (fig. 16) towards a surface. Bend your leg down wards and in the same time hold your upper body in a fix position. If you tip your back backwards you can feel even more stretch, but doing that it can strain your foot arch. It is important to use a soft surface, like a sofa or a bed. All power from the thigh is held up by the foot joint. Make sure that you really feel those muscles relax. This is essential for beneficial results in the end. Stretching one leg at a time works more smoothly.

Stretch time
1 – 3 minutes for each leg.

Your stretch time has to do with your stress level and your normal muscle tonus. This first stretch exercise demands most attention, because the size of the muscles. Make sure that you really loosing up your thigh muscles and the time your spare on this first stretch you get back in relaxing abilities and better sleep.

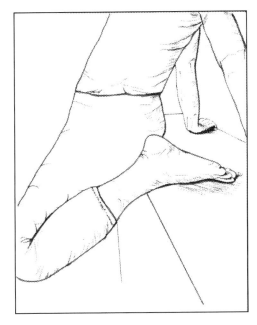

Important!

Make sure that you apply your foot on a soft surface, like a sofa or a bed.

Bend your leg down wards and in the same time decrease the angle between foot and lower leg, to protect your foot arch.

To help your foot joint, apply something soft just before the ankle, like a small folded towel or something similar.

Figure 15. Thigh stretch protection

This first exercise you can do while looking at TV. But remember, stretching is for the moment. Don't be afraid if your legs start to "sleep." Take it easy for a while and continue. You can relax in different ways: standing, sitting, or lying down. It is more convenient and practical if you sit. In a sitting position, you can use your own body weight to balance the strong leg muscles. But if you have any problem with your feet, don't do both legs. When you get to the point where you are stretching both legs at the same time, the relaxation process becomes faster, and in my opinion, it feels much better. To do the both legs at same time require really soft surface, like a sofa or a bed.

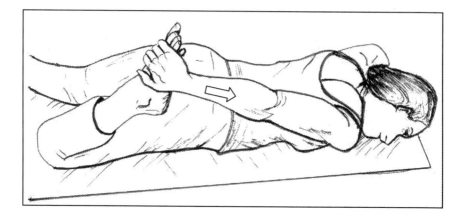

Figure 16. Alternative thigh stretch

This is an alternative thigh stretch which you can use if the first stretch exercise isn't for you. Although, you have to pull all power yourself to make the stretch, which can be quite a task. My opinion is; you can't relax, totally, at the same time you practice a muscle labor. Anyway, can't you for some reason not practice my posture try this one Instead.

Well done! The first part is finished, and you can now continue with S2S-2.

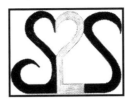

S2S-2: Calves

M. Gastrocnemius and M. Soleus

The first part of the S2S program is explaining the most essential muscles to stretch to gain the best relaxation. To gain overall good sleep, you need an arsenal of different solutions. But it's a good start to have a relaxed body, and for some, that is all they need to get a good night's sleep. Remember, you can feel different relaxation from evening to evening and from different muscle groups.

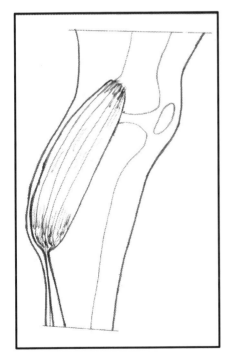

Function:

M. Gastrocnemius stretches the ankle of the foot and bends the knee.

Tense muscles give:

- Cramp in the muscle
- Problems with Achilles tendon
- Pain in arch of the foot
- Restless legs-like symptoms

Figure 17. M. Gastrocnemius

When working with the S2S program, you gain an overall health benefit. Just keep going. Before continuing with the back of the femoris, go to the lower leg. Your calf M. gastrocnemius, among other muscles, is important for relaxation. Remember, despite its size, this is a very strong muscle, one of the strongest, and it's built to take strong forces and to work a long time.

M. Gastrocnemius

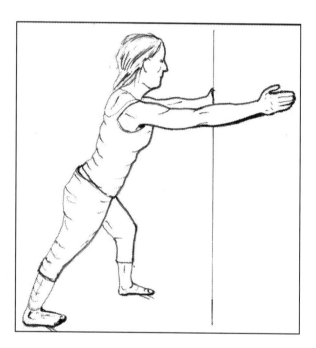

Figure 18. M. Gastrocnemius stretch

Implementation

Lean toward and put your hands against a wall. Your leg angle determines your stretch. The more you lean over toward the wall, the better effect on the calf muscle. Make sure you have your leg and torso in the same line. You will feel a nice stretch in the whole legs, but above all in M. Gastrocnemius.

This is an important exercise.

Your response to this program can be not only a notable relaxation, but other signs as well, such as a gurgling sound from the bowels. At this stage, your second exercise, you can already notice some relaxing feelings spreading in your body, and the first yawning appears suddenly. A good sign!

M. Soleus

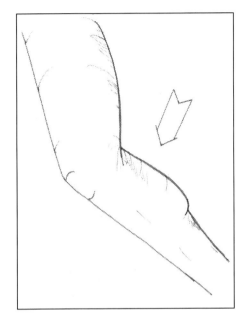

Implementation

Lean forward as in the first exercise for M. Gastrocnemius. Because this muscle is attached under your knee, you determine the angle by bending your leg downward. Your knee goes straight down, and you will sense a stretch in a very small spot of the lower leg.

Figure 19. M. Soleus stretch

Stretch time

1 – 3 minutes on each leg.

RLS Syndrome

Relaxing these muscles can be extremely beneficial in making light RLS symptoms disappear. The creeping ache from these tight muscles can be very disturbing in the beginning of the night and make it impossible to sleep. Because of this problem, these muscles cannot participate in shifting the NS. The muscle conditions in your calves are in some part responsible for your problems. RLS-type symptoms show when the calf muscles tend to tighten up and are very stiff; this should not be confused with cramping. Although not all sleep sufferers have trouble with these symptoms, they are very common.

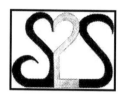

S2S-3: Back of Thigh

M. Ischio Crurales, more popularly called Hamstring

After stretching the calf muscles, we continue with the back of the thighs, or the hamstrings. This is also a strong bunch of muscles that needs some effort to loosen up.

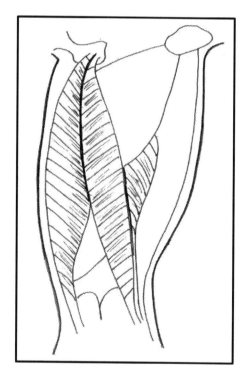

Function:

To bend the knee joint, stretch the hip joint.

Tense muscles give:

- Pain in the lower back
- Problems bending forward
- Difficulties walking or running

Figure 20. Hamstring

You have gained some overall stretching when working with the calves in the previous exercise. Remember, all stretching exercises usually affect several different muscles, not only the muscle you want to improve.

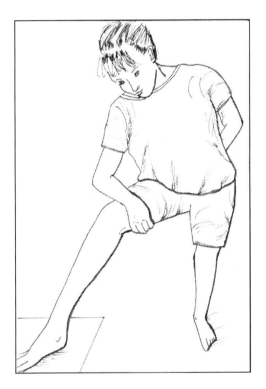

Figure 21. Back thigh stretch

Implementation

Put your foot on a sofa or stool; make sure that you have an angle of forty-five degrees from your upper to your lower leg. Lean over the leg and stretch the back of that leg. You should feel a really sharp stretch on your upper leg, and nothing from the lower part. This is an exercise that you don't need to have any doubt about. Nothing can happen, except loosening up. It's a bunch of strong muscles; have some patience. Just bend forward and try to relax, which does the trick.

Stretch time
1 – 3 minutes on each leg

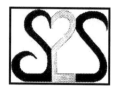

S2S-4: Back of Leg

S2S-2 and S2S-3 have already done some loosening up for the improvement of the back of your leg, so this exercise is just a combination between those two pushed further. An overall back leg stretch exercise can be a little rough, so take it easy to start with.

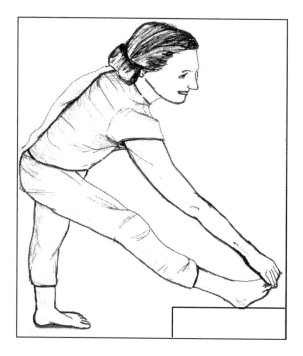

Implementation

Normally you practice this exercise with a straight leg and get a stretch in the calf and thigh. Stand up, put your leg on a bed or sofa, lean forward, and stretch. Try to grab your toe and push it down. Now the whole back of your leg should be

Figure 22. Back of leg stretch

From my point of view, we don't have to do every stretch by the book; the most important thing is that you feel a stretch and that you are working toward relief.

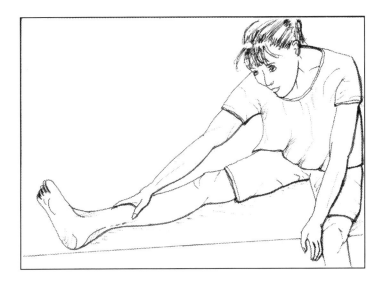

Figure 23. Alterative back of leg stretch

The benefit from this exercise is the same as from the previous two exercises. Remember, you don't know which stretch will give you the most benefits until you perform them. One evening, you might have a big yawn from a movement or exercise that didn't have any effect the previous evening. You can't be sure what exercise is best for the moment. But the combination of these exercises is for sure a great benefit.

Stretch time

1 -3 minutes on each leg

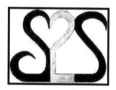

S2S-5: BOTTOM

M. Gluteus: Maximus, Medius, and Minimus

Continue to the last stretch on your lower body. This exercise is important for your sleep and most valuable for your hips.

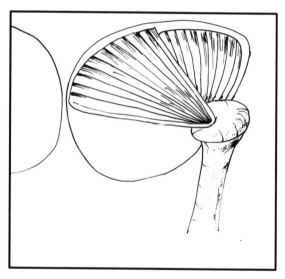

Figure 24. M. Gluteus

Function

Stretching the M. Gluteus stretches and bends the hip joint. The muscles function as stabilization for the lower back, stretching the hip joint, rotating legs, and reducing swank.

A tense muscle gives pain in:

- The lower back
- The back of the thigh
- The lateral side of the legs

Be aware that if you have any form of problem in your hips, take it easy. But a lot of pain in the hip region can sometimes have to do with a very tense M. Gluteus or muscles nearby. If you never do any form of stretching in your life, many muscles through your body can reach a spastic tone. This region also has strong muscles, so some amount of power might be needed. Use a slow movement—no jerky action.

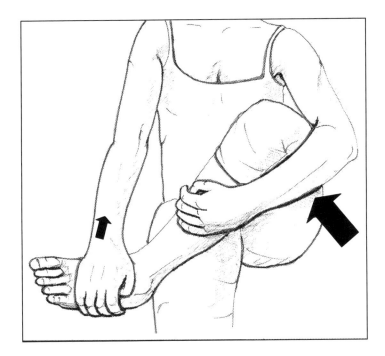

Figure 25. M. Gluteus stretch

The gluteus muscles are very strong and it will demand some effort to stretch them. I find above posture efficient enough to make the trick. If you sit like in the figure you have the opportunity to use your whole right arm to bend your leg, towards others side, as the arrow show.

OBS! With your left arm; use just a fractions of the force and maintain only the balance of the stretching exercise. Anyway, use minimal force with the left arm until you are sure about your strength of your knee joints. Normally, your knee joint is a very strong unit and can on take quit some force.

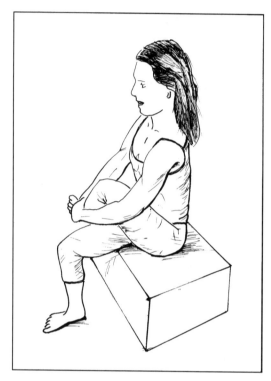

Figure 26. Alternative M. Gluteus stretch

Implementation

Sit down or you can even do it in laying down position. Bend knee toward your torso, and you get a stretch to the M. Gluteus maximus. But if you bend the knee to the same side, you get a stretch to the M. Gluteus medius and minimus. Depending on the angle, the height, and the hips, you activate different muscles. Variation and practice will teach you how to do it.

Stretch time

1 – 3 minutes on each side

End of First Part

These five basic exercises have been very useful for me through the years. I have been practicing them more or less since the beginning of the 1990s, although at that point, I didn't have any deep sense of what I was doing and I'm not sure how many exercises I started with. You might say, or feel, that it's far too easy and it can't be working. And I must be honest with you: sleep is a very complicated subject and everybody has special needs, so this might not be the only thing you have to try. Look, why not get started? My hope is that the S2S program could be one piece of an answer to your sleep puzzle needs. What I have shown so far are the most beneficial exercises to support onset of sleep. I also believe you can gain an overall positive effect from them, not only better sleep quality. I know that a lot of people are doing stretching exercises or yoga. But the key issue is the time factor. If you are doing exercise after your workout or in the morning, it's not beneficial for your sleep in a major way because, as I described earlier, stretching is for the moment; you cannot store relaxation. When you want to get tension relief, for instance, when going to bed at night, do these exercises. Sometimes I fool myself and do not do any stretching, but in the morning, I almost always know that I didn't sleep as I should have. If you don't want to continue with more exercises, it's all right, but I have a few more that have overall benefits. Now, we have been working with the lower part of the body, and it's time to gain some relaxation in the upper part. Although the upper part is not that important for sleep benefit, there are some key areas that need to be looked after that is essential in daily life. I will show you some exercises for your shoulders, neck, and arms. These exercises may have a big impact when doing your daily routine. Whenever you are sitting, standing, or working at work, whatever you do can give you a reminder in the form of pain or aches. While the lower parts just get stiff, the upper region can get tense pretty fast, and if you don't pay attention to the signs, it can get worse. Computer work is sedentary work, and it's easy to get over tense muscles or joints. Stretching those parts can make you feel ready the next workday and help you gain better sleeping skills, as well. Still, you cannot compare the efficiency of these exercises to those for the lower parts of your body.

If you just have 10 min to spare, make this first part as yours;

10 minutes stretch-program

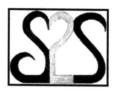

S2S-6: Neck

M. Trapezius and M. Suboccipitalis

After doing the above exercises, you should now have a nice release in your lower body, which was my purpose. Maybe you already have deep yawns spreading around your face, or gurgling sounds from your bowels. The lower body has the most impact on changing the nervous system.

M. Trapezius

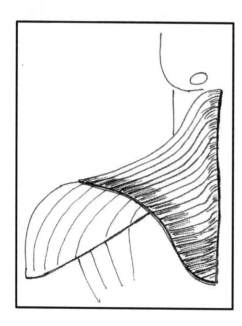

Figure 27. M. Trapezius

Functions

The M. Trapezius raises and lowers the scapula, pushing the scapula together and rotating and leaning the head aside.

A tense muscle gives:

- Headache in the base of the skull and behind the ears
- Pain above the scapula
- Difficulties leaning

Implementation

You can stand or sit when doing this exercise. It is important to maintain the shoulder in a fixed position; otherwise it is easy for the shoulders to follow the movement, and then they don't get a proper stretch. To help them stabilize; take a firm grip with that side hand (stretching side) on something where you can get a natural stop, for example, on the edge of a stole. Take your opposite hand around your head to that side ear and very gently stretch to the other side.

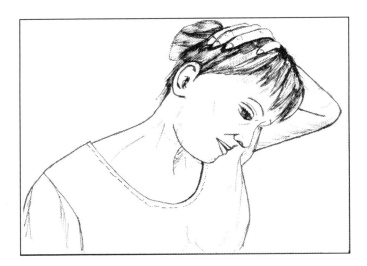

Figure 28. M. Trapezius stretch

Neck muscles are one of the many common complaint areas, and they give a nice response when exercised. Although there are a bunch of muscles supporting the head to consider when stretching, it is not very important to split them up; just do the stretch. M. Trapezius is the biggest muscle in this area; therefore, you get the most from relaxing this muscle.

Stretch time
Half a minute on each side

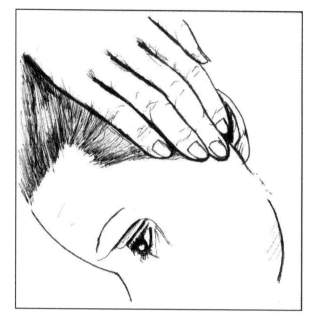

If you want a firmer grip on your head; place a fingertip in your ear, which will give you better attachment. You can feel a stronger stretch right away.

Figure 29. Alternative neck stretch

M. Trapezius is a relatively big muscle, reaching over the neck, shoulders, and top part of the back. This muscle can be tense during a stressful event when, for example, you squeeze your shoulders together.

M. Suboccipitalis

This part of the neck can be very painful during stressful events. It supports and tightens the head and the neck together. It is a group of small muscles holding the first cervical vertebrae.

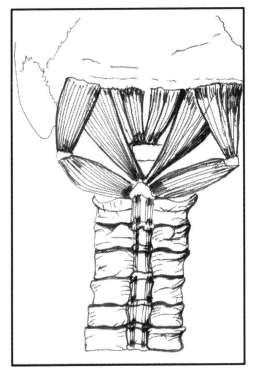

Functions

These are small muscles on the base of the skull for bending the head backward and stabilizing the head and fine motor movement.

Tense muscles give:

- Headache around the base of the skull and on top of the skull.

You can feel tens in these small muscles almost imminently in the beginning of a stressful event.

Figure 30. M. Suboccipitalis

With this exercise I use to practice both stretch and muscle work. Only because I feel this is quite a neglected part of my body. You are almost always tens in this area, mostly because of daily stressful events. We can have rather stiff neck muscles just through stress and a stiff muscle is not the same as a strong muscle. In this case is convenient to practice stretch and muscle labor at the same time.

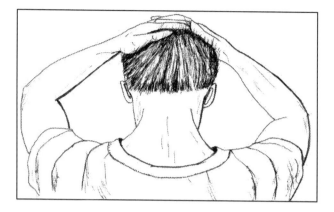

Figure 31. Suboccipitalis stretch from back

Implementation

Take a grip on the back of your head with both your hands together. Start to pull your head downwards towards your chest, with a slow motion. Then go back upwards again only with the weight of your hands and arms or without them. Don't use extra force to start with. Just repeat the move.

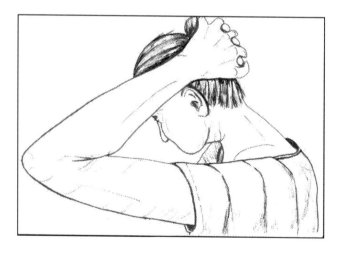

Stretch time
Half a minute

Figure 32. Suboccipitalis stretch from side

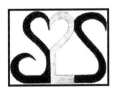

S2S- 7: Shoulder

M. Deltoideus and M. Infraspinatus

M. Deltoideus

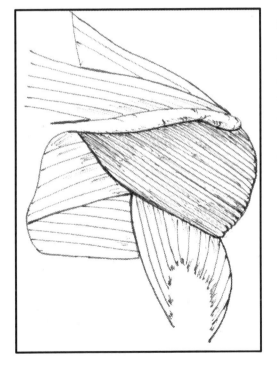

Functions:

This muscle supports direction upward, for example, lifting your arm above your head.

A tense muscle gives:

- Sore shoulders
- Cramps in muscles
- Cramps in neck joints
- Pain in arm or hands

Figure 33. M. Deltoideus

Sometimes you can feel pain and have trouble raising your arm. This condition can be chronic and can go on for years. Static work, for instance, writing at computers, can give problems in the whole arm and neck area.

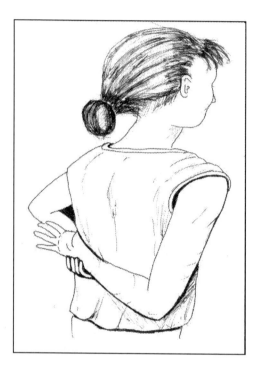

Implementation

Stand with your arms stretched. Place one arm behind your back. Use the other arm to pull the original arm toward the other side.

Figure 34. M. Deltoideus stretch

Stretch time

Half a minute on each arm

M. Infraspinatus

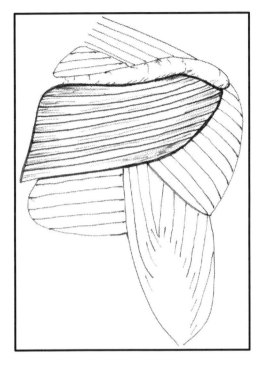

Functions:

This muscle support outward rotation and moving your arm aside.

A tense muscle gives:

- Severe pain in the front of your shoulder.

Figure 35. M. Infraspinatus

Implementation

Stand or sit. Hold your arm at a ninety-degree angle from your body, with the same angle in your elbow joint. Grip your elbow with your other hand and stretch the elbow toward the other shoulder.

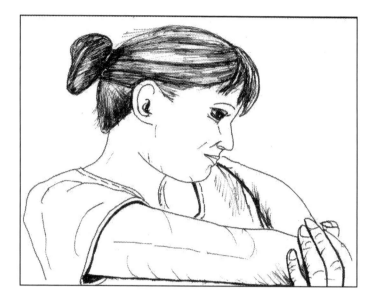

Figure 36. M. Infraspinatus stretch

To Think About

When you have pain in the front of your shoulder, try to find a sore point in the middle of the M. Infraspinatus; this is a trigger point at the whole front of the shoulder. Ask a friend to help you with hard massage of that area. If you find the right spot, you can apply strong force without any harm, but do not apply the force except just over this spot.

Stretch time
Half a minute on each arm

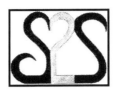

S2S-8: Lower Arm
M. Extensors/M. Brachioradialis and M. Flexors

M. Brachioradialis

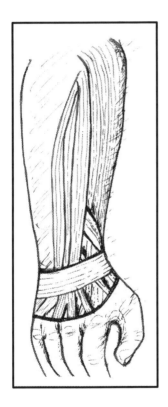

M. Extensors of the Lower Arm

These are several small muscles on the "outside" of the lower arm.

Function

They extend and abduct the hand at the wrist.

This muscle often demonstrated its weakness when playing tennis, and therefore it got the name "tennis elbow." Whatever you do, especially if you work with your hands, it is important to stretch this part. It can also be important for your sleep.

Figure 37 M. Brachioradialis

In the last exercise, we concentrated on the lower arm. I do this exercise because I know it's beneficial for the overall health of the elbow and wrist.

Exercising this muscle will not give major results for your sleep, but in our modern world of, for instance, computer work, it's a great move.

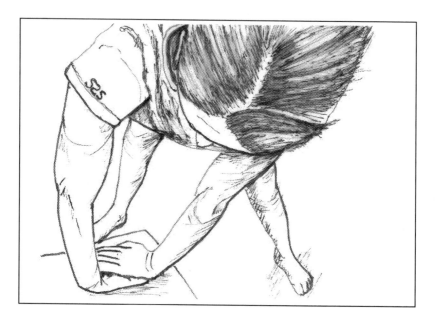

Figure 38. M. Brachioradialis stretch

Implementation

Use a soft surface, a sofa or a bed.

These muscles are small and therefore easy to work with. When you want to stretch M. Brachioradialis, you do the same, with the difference; you bending arm outwards. Right away, you feel a stretch from your elbow to your hand.

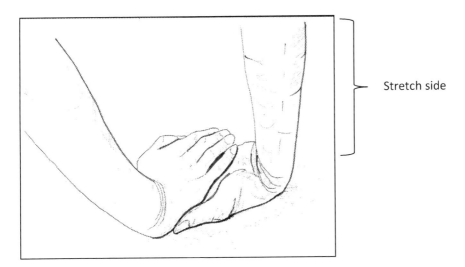

Stretch side

Figure 39. M. Brachioradialis stretch

Stretch time
Half a minute on each arm

Just take it easy, if this is the first time you practice this move. To make sure you don't harm the junction of hand and arm.

M. Flexors of the lower Arm

M. Flexors are several small muscles on the "inside" of your lower arm.

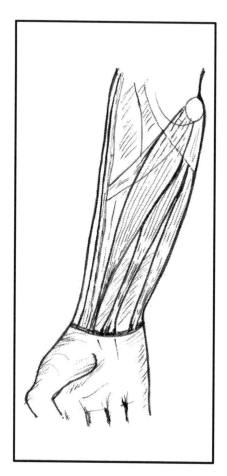

Functions:

Pronation and flexion of the forearm, and flexes and adducts the anterior of the wrist joint.

Anything you do, for example, gripping a handle for some purpose, it can give pain in the end. Now, if M. Brachioradialis gave you trouble when playing tennis, this muscle has a different weak sport—golf.

The grip of the club and the swing can give pain in the area of the elbow, and this is therefore named golf elbow. A little stretching and massage can greatly help the sore muscle and tendon.

Figure 40. M. Flexors

Implementation

Practice like in Figure 46. Use a soft surface, like a bed or a sofa. Be a little careful if you're doing it for the first time.

When I stretch this part, I think the flexors are harder than the extensors. It can feel different from person to person, of course.

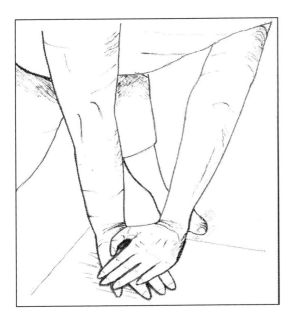

Figure 41. M. Flexors stretch

Stretch time
Half a minute on each arm

Conclusion

That was it! It might be a mountain to climb, you think. But I can assure you that this is really easy to get to a routine pretty quickly. If you feel the whole stretching program is too much, do only the first part, which is really important! The legs can easily become stiff, and you know how that can interfere with your sleep quality. With my S2S program, I want to share what I have been doing for many years. I still follow this program. I promise you, I'll never quit. I said it before: you cannot relax your muscles mentally. At least now you have a technique to use whenever you want.

I'm not going to fool you. Unfortunately, this is not the only truth to promote good sleep, but this is only a couple pieces of the sleep puzzle. But why not have a couple more of those precious pieces?

Do these exercises properly, and you'll feel the difference.

I never had any negative experiences myself practicing S2S-program, but everybody is unique and therefore should be practicing according to their own skills and experience, after a while you get your own technique. But, if you don't have any physical experience before, take it easy to start with. You can't be too careful.

And the last comments come from my twin brother. He said, not long ago; "I be angry if I forget or been lazy not to practice the S2S-Program every evening, because I can feel it's very beneficial for my sleep and body". Good comments brother.

I wish you a wonderful night and a restful wake up.

GOOD LUCK!

Index

References

A

Aagaard P, Magnusson P S, Larsson B, Kjær M and Krustrup P; *Mechanical Muscle Function, Morphology, and Fiber Type in Lifelong Trained Elderly; Posted 11/16/2007. Medicine and Science in Sports and Exercise. 2007. 39(11):1989 1996. 2007 American College of Sports Medicine*

Allen R P; *Uncovering the need to sleep. Case studies on management of restless legs syndrome; Scientific presentation; http//208.40.175.32/cecity/Flash App/ prime /restless leg/print.pdf*

Anderson P; *Significant Changes in Sleep Pattern Can Affect Mortality Risk; Journalist Medscape; Medcape Medical New*

Aserinsky E and Kleitman N; *Two types of ocular motility occurring in sleep; J Appl. Physiol. Jul 1955; 8 (1):1–10.*

http://www.askdrsears.com/topics/sleep-problems/8-infant-sleep-facts-every-parent-should-know

B

Barclay L; *Muscular Strength in Men Linked to Lower All-Cause and cancer mortality; Medscape Medical News*

Barclay L; *Qigong, Exercise therapy Effective for long-term, non specific neck pain; Medscape Medical News*

Barclay L; *Reactions to Stress May Affect Brain Aging; Medscape Medical News*

Barclay L; *Short sleep duration linked to cardiovascular risk in patients with hypertension; Medscape Medical News*

Barclay L, Author Charles Vega; Strength and Endurance Exercises Decrease; Chronic Neck Pain; Medscape News

Basheer R, Strecker RE, Thakkar M and McCarley R W; Adenosine and sleep-wake regulation; Prog. Neurobiol. 73 (6): 379–96.

Bello-Hass V D, Florence J M, Kloos A D, Scheirbecker J, Lopate G, Hayes S M. Pioro E P and Mitsumoto H; A randomized controlled trial of resistance exercise in individuals ALS. Neurology 2007 Jun 5. 68(23)2003-7

Benbadis S R, Professor, Director of Comprehensive Epilepsy Program, Departments of Neurology and Neurosurgery, University of South Florida School of Medicine, Tampa General Hospital; Normal Sleep EEG; Medscape

Benca R; the Impact of Stress on Insomnia and Treatment Considerations, Professor, Department of Psychiatry, University of Wisconsin – Madison; From Medscape Neurology > Insomnia and Sleep Health Expert Column

Benington J H and Heller H C; Progress in Neurobiology; Vol. 45 pp 347-360. 1995; Elsevier Science Ltd. Printed in Great Britain. 0301-0082/95

Benloucif S., Guico M J, Reid K J and Wolfe L F L'hermite-Balériaux M and Zee P C; Stability of melatonin and temperature as circadian phase markers and their relation to sleep times in humans; Journal of Biological Rhythms 20 (2): 178–88. April 2005

Berg K; Den stora Stretchboken; Fitness förlaget, 2004

Bethesda; Post-exercise Caffeine helps muscles refuel; http://www.the-aps.org/mm/hp/Audiences/Public-Press/For-the-Press/releases/Archive/ 08/24.html

Bienenfeld D, Professor of Psychiatry, Vice-Chair and Director of Residency Training, Department of Psychiatry, Wright State University, Boonshoft School of Medicine; Parasomnia; Chief Editor: Stephen Soreff, MD President of Education Initiatives, Nottingham, NH; Faculty, Metropolitan College of Boston University, Boston, Ma

Bonati MT, Ferini-Strambi L and Aridon P et al; Autosomal dominant restless legs syndrome maps on chromosome 14q; Brain 2003; 126:1485–92

Brown A J; Restless Leg Syndrome More Common Than Previously Thought; From Reuters Health Information

Busse E and Busse P; Akupunktur-Fibel, Die Praxis der Chinesichen Akupunkturlehre; Richard Phlaum Verlag München

C

Cheng B, Anea C B, Yao L, Chen F, Patel V, Merloiu A, Pati P, Caldwell R W, Fulton D J and Rudic R D; Tissue-intrinsic dysfunction of circadian clock confers transplant arteriosclerosis; http://www.pnas.org/content/ 108/41/ 17147; 2011

Childs J D, Cleland J A, Elliott L M, Teyhen D S, Godges J and Flynn T W; Neck Pain: Clinical Practice Guidelines Linked to the International Classification of Functioning, Disability, and Health From the Orthopaedic Section of the American Physical Therapy Association; J Orthop. Sports Phys Ther 2008:38(9):A1-A34.

Chopra Deepak, MD; God Sömn; Translation Kristina Larsén from Restful Sleep; Scandbook AB, Falun 1998

Colrain M, Crowley K E, Nicholas C L, Afifi L, Baker F and Padilla C, et al.; Sleep evoked delta frequency responses show a linear decline in amplitude across the adult lifespan; Neurobiology of Aging, 31(5), 874-883, 2010

Crick, Mitchison and Graeme; The function of dream sleep; Nature 304 (5922): 111–114. 1983

Charles A and Czeisler C A, PhD, MD Harvard Medical School and Brigham and Women's Hospital Boston, MA; Sleeping Better in Space: Sleep Studies and Clinical Trials of Melatonin as a Hypnotic

Czisch M, Dresler M, Koch S P, Wehrle R, Spoormaker V I, Holsboer F, Stieger A and Sämann P G, Obrig H; Dreamed Movement Elicits Activations in the Sensormotor Cortex; Current Biology, 21(21)pp. 1833-1837, 2011

D

Dang-Vu T, McKinney S M, Buxton O M, Solet J M and Ellenbogen J M; Spontaneous brain rhythms predict sleep stability in the face of noise; Current Biology, 10 August 2010, Vol. 20, Issue 15, pp. R626-R627

Dement W C and Vaughan C; The promise of sleep: a pioneer in sleep medicine explores the vital connection between health, happiness, and a good night's sleep; New York: Delacorte Press. 1999

Dimsdale J E, MD; Psychological Stress and Cardiovascular Disease; Medscape News

Djousse L and Gaziano J M; Alcohol use may cut risk of heart failure with hypertension; Harvard Medical School, Boston; the American Journal o Cardiology; 2008, 102: 593–597

F

FAQ Statistical Yearbook 2004 Vol. 1/1 Table C.10: Most important imports and exports of agricultural products; http://fao.org/statstics/yearbook

Fisone G, Borgkvist A and Usiello A (April 2004); Caffeine as a psychomotor stimulant: mechanism of action; Cell. Mol. Life Sci. 61 (7–8): 857–72.

Freedman N D, Park Y, Abnet C, Hollenbeck A R, and Sinha R; Association of Coffee Drinking with Total and Cause-Specific Mortality; N Engl. J Med 2012; 366:1891–1904; May 17, 2012

Freeman Morgillo S, PhD; Cognitive Behavioral Therapy in Advanced Practice Nursing: An Overview; Medscape

Friedman, Howard S.; Booth-Kewley, Stephanie; Personality, Type A behavior, and coronary heart disease: The role of emotional expression. Journal of Personality and Social Psychology, Vol 53(4), Oct 1987, 783–792.

G

Garfinkel M, EdD; Yoga as a Complementary Therapy; http://walteryogatherapy blogspot.se/2008/02/yoga-as-complementary-therapy.html

Garodia P, Ichikawa H, Malani N, Sethi G and Aggarwal BB; From ancient medicine to modern medicine: ayurvedic concepts of health and their role in inflammation and cancer; The University of Texas M. D. Anderson Cancer Center, Houston, TX; J Soc Integr Oncol. 2007. Winter; 5(1):25–37.

Graeber R C 1, Rosekind M R 1, Connell L J 1 and Dinges D F 2; 1. Cockpit Napping Flight Human Factors Branch; NSA Ames Research Center 2 Institute of Pennsylvania Hospital; University of Pennsylvania School of Medicine

Griffin J, Tyrrell I; Dreaming Reality: how dreaming keeps us sane or can drive us mad; Human Givens Publishing. 2004

H

Hannan L M, Jacobs E J and Thun M J; Smoking and Risk of Colorectal Cancer in Large Prospective Cohort from United States; Cancer Epidemiology, Biomarkers & Prevention; http//cebp.aecrjournals.org/content/18/12/ 3362.full

Haskell W L, Lee I-M; Russell R P, Powell K E, Blair S N, Franklin B A, Macera C A; Heath G W, Thompson P D and Bauman A; Physical Activity and Public Health: Updated Recommendation for Adults; From the American College of Sports Medicine and the American Heart Association

Hening W A and Montplaisir J; Insights In to Restless Legs Syndrome: Understanding the Patient Experience to Improve Outcomes (Slides with Transcript); Medscape

Insomnia and *Stretch to Sleep*™-Program

Henry J A, Professor, Chief Medical Editor; New Guide to Medicines & Drugs; The British Medical Association; A Dorling Kindersley Book

Herthz G, Director, Center for Insomnia and Sleep Disorder, Clinical Associate Professor of Psychiatry and Behavioral Sciences, State University of New York at Stony Brook; Sleep Dysfunction in women; Medscape

Hobson J A; The Dream Drugstore: Chemically Altered State of Consciousness; Hardcover, Paperback

Horne J A and Östberg O; A self-assessment questionnaire to determine morningness-eveningness in human circadian rhythms; Int. J Chronobiol 4 (2): 97–110. 1976

Hughes S; Regular Exercise Can Help Preserve/Build Heart Mass; Exercise and heart mass; Heartwire

Humphrey N; Dreaming as play; Centre for Philosophy of Natural and Social Sciences; London School of Economics, London WC2A, United Kingdom

Huss M; Alcoholismus chronicus: Stockholm und Leipzig, 1852, Retrieved 19 February 2008; http//:books.google.com/ ?id= wt62Z w8sCEC&pg=PR5

I

The International Classification of Sleep Disorders, Revised: Diagnostic and Coding Manuel. 2001 edition. Library of Congress Catalog No. 97-71405, 2001 Retrieved 2010-08-08

IRLSSG, International Restless Legs Syndrome Study Group, C. General aspects of dream psychology. In: Dreams. Princeton, NJ: Princeton University Press, 23–66 1948. ;http: //irlssg.org/rls-factJung

J

Jülke W; Hälsa, Bot och Bättring; Liber Tryck Stockholm 1984

K

Kedlaya D, Clinical Associate Professor; Department of Physical Medicine and Rehabilitation, Loma Linda University School of Medicine; Postexercise muscle soreness; Medscape

L

Latham N K, Anderson C S, Reid I R; Effects of Vitamin D Supplementation on Strength, Physical Performance, and Falls in Older Persons: A Systematic Review; Medscape

Latorre J; Research Fellow, Department of Physical Medicine and Spinal Cord Injury Medicine; The Institute for Rehabilitation and Research; Restless legs Syndrome; Medscape

Lavigne G J and Montplaisir J Y; Restless legs syndrome and sleep bruxism: prevalence and association among Canadians: Sleep. 1994: 17739-73

Linton S J; Does work stress predict insomnia? A prospective study; Br J Health Psychol. 2004; 9: 127–136.

Little L, Freelance writer for Medscape; Mental Stress-Associated Blood Pressure Rise Linked to Increase in Creatinine

Loomis A L, Harvey E N, Hobart G A. Cerebral states during sleep as studies by human brain potentials. J Exp Psychol 1937; 21:127–44

Loudon A 1, Ray D 2, Meng Q J1, McMaster A 1, 2, Beesley S 1, Lu W Q 1, Gibbs J 1, Parks D3 Collins J 3, Farrow S 4, Donn R 1, 2; Ligand Modulation of REV-ERBα Function Resets the Peripheral Circadian Clock In a PhasicMmanner; 1. Faculty of Life Sciences, Manchester, UK; 2. Medical and Human Sciences, Manchester, UK; 3. GlaxoSmithKline, Research Triangle Park, USA; 4. GlaxoSmithKline, Discovery Biology, Respiratory CEDD, GSK Medicines Research Centre, Gunnels Wood Road, Stevenage SG1 2NY, UK; doi: 10.1242/jcs.035048 November 1, 2008

Lowry F; Insufficient Sleep Thwarts Weight Loss Efforts; Medscape Medical News

Lubit R H; Assistant Clinical Professor, Mount Sinai School of Medicine, New York University School of Medicine; Sleep Disorder; Medscape

Lucas M; Epidemiologist/nutritionist at Harvard School of Public Health in Boston, Massachusetts; Publ. in September 26 (2011) issue of the Archives of Internal Medicine

M

Malliaropoulos N, Papalexandris S and Papalada A, et al.. The role of stretching in rehabilitation of hamstring injuries: 80 athletes follow-up. Med Sci, Sports Exerc 2004; 36:756–9.

Malory M; The Reverse Learning Theory of Dreams; http://www.meaningofdreams. org /dream_theory/ reverselearningtheorydreams.htm

Manzoni G M, Pagnini F, Castelnuovo G and Molinari E; Relaxation Training for Anxiety: A Ten-Years Systematic Review With Meta-Analysis; Posted 07/07/2008, BMC Psychiatry

Martikainen K, Partinen M, Hasan J, Laippala P, Urponen H and Vuori I; The impact of somatic health problems on insomnia in middle age. Sleep Med. 2003; 4: 201–206.

McManama Aukerman M, Aukerman D, Bayard M, Tudiver F, Thorp L and Bailey B; Exercise and Restless Legs Syndrome: A randomized control Trial; Posted: 10/20/2006; Journal of the American Board of Family Medicine; 19(5):487–493

Melchart D, Weidenhammer W, Streng A, Hoppe A, Pfaffenrath V and Linde K; Acupuncture for Chronic Headaches – An Epidemiological Study; Posted 05/02/2006; Headache 46(4):632–641

Melody R and Slevin J T; Restless Legs Syndrome; Posted: 09/14/2006; American Journal of Health-System Pharmacy 2006; 63 17: 1599–1612. 2006 American Society of Health-System Pharmacists

MHRA; Medicine and Healthcare products Regulatory Agency http:// www.mhra.gov.uk/ home/groups/pl-p/documents/ websiteresources/ con 2024428.pdf

Mills E, Wu P, Seely D and Guyatt G; November 2005); Melatonin in the treatment of cancer: a systematic review of randomized controlled trials and meta-analysis". J. Pineal Res. 39 (4): 360–6. Nov 2005.

http://www.cdc.gov/MMWR/preview/mmwrhtml/mm5206a2.htm

Montplaisir J, Philips B A and Lee H B; Restless Legs Syndrome: Impact, Recognition, and Management (Slides with Transcript); Medscape

N

NCB/ULF; Statistics Sweden; http://www.scb.se/Pages/Product12199.aspx

http://nccam.nih.gov/news/camstats/2007/camsurvey_fs1.htm; How Many People Use CAM

Nelson K R; American Academy of Neurology; People with near Death Experiences can differ in sleep-wake control; The Journal of Neurology; Released April 10 2006

NIH Publication; US Department of Health and Human Services; National Institutes of Health; National Heart, Lung and Blood Institute; NIH Publication No. 06-5271; November 2005

Ninivaggi F J, Associate Attending Physician at Yale-New Haven Hospital, Assistant Clinical Professor of Child Psychiatry at Yale University School of Medicine; 1. An Elementary Textbook of Ayurveda: Medicine with a Six Thousand Year Old Tradition, Psychosocial Press, 2001; 2. Ayurveda: A Comprehensive Guide to Traditional Indian Medicine for the West, Rowman & Littlefield Publishers Inc, 2010.

NSF, National Sleep Foundation; Reviewed by Michael V Viteillo, PhD; Associate Director of the Northwest Geriatric Education Center and a Professor of Psychiatry

Insomnia and *Stretch to Sleep™*-Program

and Behavioral Sciences http:// www.sleepfoundation.org/ article/sleep-topics/aging-and-sleep

O

Oto A, Aykac O, Yilmaz N and Akbostanci M C, Prevalence of restless legs syndrome in Ankara, Turkey (abstract); Movement Disorder 2012:27 Suppl. 1:27

P

Pandi-Perumal S, Srinivasan V, Poeggeler B, Hardeland R and Cardinali D P; Drug Insight: The Use of Melatonergic Agonists for the Treatment of Insomnia -- Focus on Ramelteon; Nat Clin Pract Neurol. 2007;3(4):221-228. © 2007 Nature Publishing Group

Passaro E A, Director, Comprehensive Epilepsy Program/Clinical Neurophysiology Lab, Bayfront Medical Center; Insomnia; Medscape

Penev P; When dieting to lose weight, how much you sleep may be as important as how much you eat; publ. in Annals of Internal Medicine; the Journal of the America College of Physicians

Peyrache A, Khamassi M, Benchenane K, Wiener S I and Battaglia F P; Replay of rule-learning related neural patterns in the prefrontal cortex during sleep; Nature Neuroscience 12 (7): 919–926. 2009

Phillips A C and Burns V E, 1 Lord J M 2; Stress and Exercise: Getting the Balance Right for Aging Immunity; 1 School of Sport and Exercise Sciences 2 Department of Immunology, University of Birmingham, Birmingham, United Kingdom

Postuma R B, Gagnon J F, Rompré S and Montplaisir J Y; Severity of REM atonia loss in idiopathic REM sleep behavior disorder predicts Parkinson disease; Department of Neurology (R.B.P.), McGill University, Montreal General Hospital, Montreal; Centre d'Etude du Sommeil et des Rythmes Biologiques (R.B.P., J.F.G., S.R., J.Y.M.), Hôpital du

Sacre-Coeur, Montreal; and Department of Psychiatry (J.F.G., J.Y.M.), Université de Montréal, Quebec, Canada.

Pray W S; Treating Sore Muscles and Tendons; Posted: 06/12/2006; US Pharmacist. 2006; 31 (5) 2006 Jobson Publishing

R

Rama A N and Kushida C A; Restless Legs Syndrome; Medscape Neurology. 2005;7 (2) http://www.medscape.org/viewarticle/511783_4

Ranjan A, MD, Palliative Medicine Physician, Associate Medical Director; Primary Insomnia; Medscape

Rapson L and Robert Banner R; Acupuncture for pain management; Geriatrics and Aging. 2008; 11(2):93-97. © 2008 1453987 Ontario, Ltd

Reese J P, Stiasny-Kolster K; Oertel W H and Dodel R C; Health-related Quality of Life and Economic Burden in Patients, with Restless Legs Syndrome; Posted: 11/28/2007; Expert Rev Pharmacoeconomics Outcomes Res. 2007;7(5):503–521. 2007. Future Drugs Ltd.

Revonsuo A, Professor, University of Skövde; School of Humanities and Informatics; The Reinterpretation of Dreams: An evolutionary hypothesis of the function of dreaming; Behavioral and Brain Sciences; 23 (6): 877–901 2000

S

Sahar S and Sassone Corsi P; Metabolism and Cancer: The Circadian Clock Connection; Posted: 03/19/2010; Nat Rev Cancer. 2009; 9(12):886–96. 2009 Nature Publishing Group

Saper C B, Fuller P M and Lu J; Differential Rescue of Light and Food-Entrainable Circadian Rhythm; Science. 2008 May 23; 320(5879):1074–7

Sarno J, Sierpina V S and Frenkel M A; Acupuncture: A Clinical Review; Posted: 04/01/2005; South Med J. 2005; 98(3):330–337. 2005 Lippincott Williams & Wilkins

Scott E; Power Napping for Increased Productivity, Stress Relief & Health, Updated March 11, 2012; http://stress.about.com/od /lowstresslifestyle/ a/ powernap.htm

See S; Regina Ginzburg, PharmD; Skeletal Muscle Relaxants; Posted: 05/22/2008; Pharmacotherapy. 2008; 28(2):207–213. 2008 Pharmacotherapy Publications

Seidman R J, Director of Neuropathology, Clinical Associate Professor, Department of Pathology, Stony Brook University Medical Center; Muscle Biopsy and the Pathology of Skeletal Muscle

Shang A; Huwiler K; Nartey L; Jüni P and Egger M; Placebo - Controlled Trials of Chinese Herbal Medicine and Conventional Medicine – Comparative Study; Posted: 12/19/2007; International Journal of Epidemiology; 36(5): 1086–1092

Sheps D S; Mental Stress May Hurt the Heart; University of Florida, posted in Journal of the American College of Cardiology

Sherin J E, Elmquist J K, Torrealba F and Saper C B; Innervation of histaminergic tuberomammillary neurons by GABAergic and galaninergic neurons in the ventrolateral preoptic nucleus of the rat; J Neurosci 18 (12): 4705–21. June 1998. http://www.jneurosci.org/cgi /content/full /18 /12 /4705

Sierpina V S and Frenkel M A; Acupuncture: A Clinical Review, Posted: 04/01/2005; South Med J. 2005; 98(3):330–337. 2005 Lippincott Williams & Wilkins

Sleep in America Poll 2003; National Sleep Foundation; website: http://www.sleepfoundation.org/sites/default/files/2003SleepPollExecSumm.pdf

Snell R S, Emeritus Professor of Anatomy, George Washington University School of Medicine and Health Sciences; Clinical Anatomy, for medical Students, Fourth Edition

Spivey A; Lose Sleep, Gain Weight: Another Piece of the Obesity Puzzle; 2010; 118(1):A28–A33. 2010 National Institute of Environmental Health Sciences

Stevens M S, University of Kansas School of Medicine, Chief Editor: Benbadis S R; Normal Sleep, Sleep Physiology, and Sleep Deprivation; http://emedicine medscape.com/article/1188226-overview

Stevenson J R and colleagues; Stopping moderate drinking may lead to depression; Neuropsychopharmacology, Published online June 18, 2008

Stranges S, Dorn J M; Shipley M J, Kandala N-B; Trevisan M; Miller M A, Donahue R P; Hovey K M; Ferrie J E, Marmot M G and Cappuccio F G; Correlates of Short and Long Sleep Duration: A Cross-Cultural Comparison Between the United Kingdom and the United States; Posted 02/20/2009; American Journal of Epidemiology; 2008; 198(11):1353–1353

Suleman A, MD, Consultant in Electrophysiology and Cardiovascular Medicine, Department of Internal Medicine, Division of Cardiology, Medical City Dallas Hospital; Exercise Prescription; Updated Sept 11 2008 http://www.tripdatabase.com/ doc/831043-Exercise-Prescription--Overview-#content

T

Tamminen J, Payne J D, Stickgold R, Wamsley E R and Gaskell G M; Sleep spindle activity is associated with the integration of new memories and existing knowledge; the Journal of Neuroscience, 30(43), 14356-60, 2010

Tanskanen A, Tuomilehto J, Viinamäki H, Vartiainen E, Lehtonen J and Puska P; Heavy coffee drinking and the risk of suicide; European Journal of Epidemiology, 2000, Volume 16, Number 9, Page 789–791

Terry N R, Medical writer and editor, Jackson Heights, New York; What Is the Attraction of Alternative Medicine; Medscape Family Medicine; Posted 09/08/2009

Terzano M G, Parrino L, Bonanni E, Cirignotta F, Ferrillo F, Luigi G and Gigli G L; Savarese M; Ferini-Strambi L; Members of the Advisory Board; Insomnia in General Practic; A consensus report produced be sleep specialist and primary-care physicians in Italy; Posted 12/22/2005

Thie J F, Doctor of Chiropractic; *Kroppsbalansering, translation from Touch for Health* by Bippan Norberg and Péter Szil

Townsend G; Ysha De Donna; *Pulses and Impulses;* Thorsons Publishing Group

U

Utsugi M, Saijo Y, Yoshioka E, et al. Relationships of occupational stress to insomnia and short sleep in Japanese workers. Sleep. 2005; 28: 728–735

V

Van Cauter E, Leproult R and Plat L.; Age-related changes in slow-wave sleep and REM sleep and relationship with growth hormone and cortisol levels in healthy men". Journal of the American Medical Association 284 (7): 861–868. 2000; doi: 10.1001/jama.284.

Vaughn McCall W; Exploring the relationship between Insomnia and Depression; Medscape

Vega C, MD, FAAFP; Acupuncture or Relaxation Training for Tension Headache: A Viewpoint; Posted 01/10/2007; Medscape Family Medicine

Vignau J, Bailly D, Duhamel A, Vervaecke P, Beuscart R and Collinet C; Epidemiologic study of sleep quality and troubles in French secondary school adolescents; J Adolesc Health. 1997: 21: 343–350

W

Wagner U, Hallschmid M, Rasch B, Born J; Brief sleep after learning keeps emotional memories alive for years. Journal: Biol. Psychiatry Year: 2006; Volume: 60. Issue: 7, Pages: 788-90

Westenbroeka C, Den Boera J A, Veenhuisb M and Ter Horsta G J; Chronic stress and social housing differentially affect neurogenesis in male and female rats; a)

Department of Psychiatry, Graduate School of Behavioral and Cognitive Neurosciences, University of Groningen, The Netherlands, b) Eukaryotic Microbiology, Groningen Biomolecular Sciences and Biotechnology Institute, University of Groningen, Netherlands

Whalen D J, Silk J S, Semel M, Forbes E E, Ryan N D, David A. Axelson, Birmaher B and Ronald E. Dahl; Caffeine Consumption, Sleep, and Affect in the Natural Environments of Depressed Youth and Healthy Controls; Oxford Journals; Journal of Pediatric Psychology, Volume 33, Issue 4, Pp 358–367

WHO; Acupuncture: Review and Analysis of Reports on Controlled Clinical Trials; http://apps.who.int/iris/bitstream/10665/42414/1/9241545437.pdf

WHO; International statistical classification of diseases and related health problems 10th ed. Geneva: The Organization; 1992

Williams J S; Depression, PTSD, Substance Abuse Increase in Wake of September 11 Attacks; National Institute of Drug Abuse, NIDA; Archives, Vol. 17 No. 4, November 2002

Wilson J; the 21st Century stress syndrome; Publ. by Smart Publications Petaluma, CA

Y

Ylinen J, Kautianinen H, Wiren K, and Kakkinen A; Stretching exercise vs manual therapy in treatment of chronic neck pain: a randomized, control cross-over trial; J Rehabil Med. 2007;39:126-132; http//dx.doi.org/10.2340/16501977-0015

Z

Zhao C-h, Stillman M J and Rozen T D, MD; Traditional and Evidence-Based Acupuncture in Headache Management: Theory, Mechanism, and Practice; Posted 07/07/2005; Headache; 45(6):716–730

All information in this book are due to my own experiences for a long period of time, but every human is unique, and therefore should be aware of theirs special needs. Don't practice anything you don't find safe or practical for you.

Find more information on S2S-movement in: **www.stretch2sleep.org**